and interpret them when convenient, thus offering more scheduling flexibility for those on both ends of the communications link. In addition to patient care, these varied technologies have a multiplicity of current and possible uses in professional education, research, public health, and administration. Such multiple uses potentially allow costs for expensive information and communications investments to be spread more broadly.

This report was prompted by the scarcity of careful evaluations of patient care applications of telemedicine. It presents a broad framework for evaluating clinical applications of telemedicine and argues for more systematic and rigorous assessments of their effects on health care quality, accessibility, costs, and acceptability compared to alternative services. For telemedicine, as for any health technology or service, such assessments are essential for several reasons. They can

- guide policymakers considering whether to encourage telemedicine by stimulating infrastructure development, funding specific telemedicine programs, or reducing policy barriers;
- provide clinicians and patients appropriate reassurance or caution about telemedicine applications;
- inform health plan managers pondering whether clinical telemedicine is feasible, cost-effective, and acceptable to patients and clinicians; and
- help those who have invested in telemedicine find ways to identify problems and improve programs.

Because telemedicine is actually a family of quite diverse technologies and applications and because important educational, research, public health, and administrative uses and benefits may be intertwined with patient care uses, the evaluation framework proposed here will have to be adapted to fit different applications and environments. It may also have to be modified to consider links to other clinical and nonclinical programs that share parts of the same technical and human infrastructure. Such modification and adaptations notwithstanding, at the heart of the evaluation framework is a body of principles and methods that form the foundation for health services research and evaluation research generally. This report attempts to relate those principles and methods to the special challenges and problems in evaluating telemedicine. It is aimed primarily at policymakers, clinicians, patients, and managers, but it should also provide context and support for researchers and evaluators with an interest in assessing information and telecommunications technologies.

TELEMEDICINE IN CONTEXT

Concerns about access to health care have propelled much of the interest in clinical applications of telemedicine. Applications have often concentrated on remote locales in the hope that they could make needed services more available to mountain families, tribal members on Indian reservations in the Southwest and the Dakotas, military personnel on tiny Pacific islands, and ranchers and others scattered across the country's open spaces. The promise has been that telemedicine could be more practical, affordable, and sustainable than traditional programs, including those intended to sustain or expand rural health care facilities and to attract physicians, nurses, and other personnel to remote areas on a short- or long-term basis. That this potential needs to be demonstrated is the thesis of this report.

Today, with the nation's health care system undergoing profound changes, telemedicine is attracting attention beyond rural areas. To the extent that telemedicine offers mechanisms for centralizing specialists, reducing costs for specialty care, and supporting primary care clinicians, managed care plans may find certain applications attractive in the urban and suburban areas they typically serve. Some academic medical centers, faced with reduced revenues and exclusion from local managed care networks, are exploring telemedicine options as they seek to develop new regional, national, and international markets for their highly specialized clinicians. Freestanding specialty groups, multiorganization medical consortia, and other entities likewise are investigating telemedicine as they seek farflung clients for their services.

The prospect of a physician surplus coupled with declining personal income has become a real concern for many physicians, particularly specialists (Pew Health Professions Commission, 1995; IOM, 1996). Nurses likewise are facing pressures from decreasing hospital utilization and a reordering of nursing practices in managed care, although these may be offset to some degree by more options in home, community, and office settings. Intense price competition is threatening the missions and even the existence of some academic health centers, public and community hospitals, community health centers, and other institutions whose costs are increased by education, research, or care for the uninsured and underinsured. In these contexts, the information and telecommunications technologies that constitute telemedicine have the potential to radically reshape health care in both positive and negative ways. In particular, over time, the widespread adoption of clinical applications of telemedicine could fundamentally alter the personal, face-to-face relationship between patient and practitioner that has been the model for medical care for generations.

Although economic considerations are stimulating many explorations of telemedicine for clinical, educational, and administrative purposes, health care organizations must also be concerned about how telemedicine could affect the actual and perceived quality of their services. As in other areas, quality assessment and improvement for telemedicine is closely linked to the continued development and implementation of sophisticated clinical, research, administrative, and other information systems.

Despite its multiplying uses and users, many forms of clinical telemedicine are still far from being routinely integrated into most facets of health care delivery. Given the scarcity of comprehensive and reliable data and the pace of change, an overall picture of telemedicine's current status must be painted in rather broad strokes. Consider, for example, the dimensions of the U.S. health system (IOM, 1992a):

Roughly 250 million patients and potential patients. Most adults have probably used the telephone to get medical advice or information. A growing number of Americans have personal computers and software that allow them to use medical databases (including some developed for clinicians or researchers rather than patients) and communicate with clinicians and others via electronic mail. An unknown, but undoubtedly tiny, fraction of the population has participated in an "electronic housecall," a video consultation with a distant medical specialist, or some other kind of interactive, audiovisual telemedicine application.

Over a half-million physicians, 1.5 million nurses, and many other health care professionals. Again, most practitioners have probably used the telephone to discuss patient care; many have participated in continuing medical education by teleconference; and some specialists such as radiologists are gaining considerable experience with the transmission of images for consultation purposes. An increasing number of clinicians have on-line access to the National Library of Medicine's Medline and other resources that allow them to search the medical literature. A growing number of health care organizations have home pages on the World Wide Web that provide information and links to information available at other sites. On-line journals are also springing up, which is raising concern about weakening of the screening and quality assurance functions served by traditional journals' peer review processes.

Thousands of hospitals, nursing homes, clinics, and other health care institutions. The number of health care institutions that have advanced telemedicine capacity (e.g., video as well as telephone and fax) is not well documented. A survey of approximately 2,400 rural hospitals conducted for the federal Office of Rural Health Policy found that nearly 20 percent reported some telemedicine services but that 60 percent reported no plans for telemedicine (Jones, 1996). Academic medical centers, community hospitals, and other institutions have created World Wide Web pages that serve both as information sources and as marketing tools. To meet internal needs and external demands, offices and hospitals are being remodeled to better accommodate information technologies that require differently configured space for people and equipment. The electronic patient record is increasingly understood to be a necessity, although practical obstacles to implementation take time to overcome.

Hundreds of managed care organizations going under a variety of acronyms, including HMOs (health maintenance organizations), PPOs (preferred providers organizations), and PHOs (physician hospital organizations). For the most part, the committee found that these organizations have more pressing priorities than telemedicine, including implementation of better patient and administrative information systems. To borrow a phrase from clinical practice, "watchful waiting" seems to be a common strategy as decisionmakers monitor the experiences of innovators and early adopters of telemedicine.

The integration of clinical, educational, and other applications of telemedicine into health care is inextricably linked to a dynamic telecommunications industry and a developing National Information Infrastructure (NII). This infrastructure has been likened to "a giant electronic web that will allow each user's computer, telephone, and television to interconnect with others, regardless of their location . . . and will enable each user to communicate with everyone else who is connected to the web" (Lasker et al., 1995). The NII has been accorded sufficient federal policy importance to be referred to by its initials as if it were a specific organization or technology rather than an evolving concept—a mix of aspirations, strategic plans, fast-changing technologies, and growing user demands and sophistication. A recent report from the National Research Council, tellingly titled *The Unpredictable Certainty: Information Infrastructure through 2000,* found that "there are as many visions of the information future as there are sectors of the economy helping to create them" (NRC, 1996, p. 3).

The technical base for telemedicine applications will also continue to be affected by innovations spurred by consumer electronics, the entertainment industry, and defense department investments. Moreover, as the telecommunications infrastructure expands to provide and support interactive educational, entertainment, retail, and other services at the "point of need" (e.g., home, school), telemedicine can be expected to follow a similar path. For example, the "electronic housecall" has the potential to save some ill or recovering patients the inconvenience or discomfort of an office visit, allow certain hospitalized patients to go home earlier, and avoid some admissions in the first instance. It may also provide preventive services to those who wish to avoid or minimize potential illness. The benefits and costs of home access to telemedicine services compared to alternative services have, however, yet to be systematically demonstrated.

Technical, clinical, organizational, and behavioral obstacles to easy use of telemedicine technologies remain, as do policy impediments and uncertainties related to reimbursement, licensure, medical liability, and other concerns. Many programs continue to depend on grants from government and industry, although some applications show more promise of becoming self-sustaining over the long term than others.

Overall, the financial and clinical justification for new or continued investment in telemedicine remains incomplete for many decisionmakers, particularly given competing demands on their resources in a period of significant economic and political uncertainty. Continued support will, in large measure, depend on better evaluation and evidence of the practicality, value, acceptability, affordability, and profitability of telemedicine.

THE DEMAND FOR EVIDENCE OF EFFECTIVENESS

Although telemedicine faces some particular challenges in the realm of evaluation, it is hardly unique in facing demands for better evidence of its effectiveness and cost-effectiveness. For more than a decade, demand has been growing for better information about the effectiveness of specific health services (OTA, 1978, 1994; Eddy, 1984; Wennberg, 1984; IOM, 1985, 1990a; 1992a; Roper et al., 1988). The commonly cited sources of this demand include the sharp escalation in health care costs during the 1970s and 1980s, the documentation of wide variations in clinical practice, the proliferation of expensive medical technologies, and the publication of studies questioning the appropriateness of a variety of health care practices.

In response, a number of public and private initiatives have been launched to extend the evidence base for health care and to improve the use of such knowledge by clinicians, patients, and other decisionmakers (see, e.g., IOM, 1985, 1990a, 1992a; Ball, 1990; PPRC, 1989; OTA, 1994). These initiatives include the establishment in 1989 of the Agency for Health Care Policy and Research, a federal agency with a specific mandate to support research, guidelines development, and other activities to increase knowledge of what works and what does not work in health care. Some medical professional organizations, including the American College of Physicians, have an even longer record of efforts to assess the effectiveness of medical services and develop evidence-based guidelines for clinical practice. Elsewhere in the private sector (often with some public funding), initiatives include research-oriented ventures such as the Medical Outcomes Trust and the Cochrane Collaboration; market-oriented enterprises such as the technology assessment collaboration of the Blue Cross and Blue Shield Association and Kaiser Permanente of Southern California; and hybrid entities such as ECRI (formerly the Emergency Care Research Institute), a nonprofit technology assessment organization in Pennsylvania.

With the proliferation of advanced and even amazing new technologies, one temptation for evaluators and decisionmakers is to focus primarily on the technical features of particular technologies and, to some degree, lose sight of clinical, administrative, educational, or other problems that they purport to address. To counter this temptation, many have urged that those devising technology assessments, guidelines for clinical practice, and similar tools start by considering clinical, organizational, and social needs and goals and then examining the benefits, risks, and costs of alternative technologies or programs within this context. This report endorses that perspective.

Most of the initiatives to improve the evidence base for health care involve both the collection and analysis of data about specific services and the development of better research tools and databases. The latter work includes efforts to

- design less expensive and more realistic methods of testing the effectiveness of alternative clinical practices;
- construct better measures of health outcomes and of care processes, delivery system characteristics, and other variables that may affect outcomes;
- devise statistical and other tools that provide more meaningful and credible analysis and presentation of data;
- build computer-based patient records and other electronic information systems that provide relatively easy and fast access to large databases and that permit the application of powerful statistical methods for analyzing and displaying those data;
- create decision support tools and learning systems that assist clinicians and patients in evaluating information, preferences, and options;
- formulate strategies for providing information to patients, clinicians, and others in ways that promote informed decisions and stimulate desired changes in behaviors and outcomes; and
- assess the effect of information and decision-support strategies on behaviors and outcomes.

Evaluations of telemedicine applications can build on these efforts as well as on a body of evaluation research concepts and methods developed in areas such as psychology, education, and welfare policy. Such evaluations can—in common with this report—likewise build on the work of a number of investigators and organizations, who have undertaken evaluations of telemedicine applications and whose contributions are reviewed in later chapters of this report.

STUDY ORIGINS AND APPROACH

The concept for this study emerged from discussions between staff of the National Library of Medicine (NLM) and the Institute of Medicine (IOM) that began in late 1994. The NLM has a long history of supporting the development of information and communications technologies to assist health researchers, clinicians, policymakers, and, increasingly, patients. For example, through Medline, Grateful Med, and Loansome Doc, the NLM has made it easier to search medical literature and find specific information for education or problem solving. The NLM has also funded a number of telemedicine demonstration projects (see Appendix A).

Although a variety of demonstration and evaluation projects have been valuable in demonstrating basic feasibility and safety, most have not been guided by a systematic framework for evaluating the impact of clinical telemedicine on the quality, accessibility, or cost of health care. Recognizing this deficiency, the National Library of Medicine (with assistance from the Health Care Financing Administration) asked the Institute of Medicine to develop a framework and related set of criteria for evaluating clinical applications of telemedicine. The evaluative focus was to be on the quality, accessibility, and cost of health care, not on technical hardware and software issues.

To undertake the requested study, the IOM appointed a 15-member committee of experts in telemedicine, medical informatics, health care delivery, health services research, quality assurance, economics, and public policy analysis. The committee met three times between July 1995 and February 1996. Staff from the NLM, the Health Care Financing Administration, the Department of Defense, the Office of Rural Health Policy of the Department of Health and Human Services, the federal Joint Working Group on Telemedicine, and other interested groups were invited to committee meetings. In addition, IOM staff and committee attended a number of meetings organized by these agencies and various private organizations.

During its deliberations, the committee identified several working principles that reflected its appreciation of the complicated and volatile state of the health care system and that shaped its examination of telemedicine and its analysis of evaluation strategies. These principles, which include a mix of practical and normative judgments or assumptions and which are one basis for the evaluation framework presented in Chapter 6, included the following:[1]

- Neither health care nor telemedicine is static.
- Systematic ways of evaluating and monitoring the impact of social, economic, and technological changes will always be needed.
- Research on the outcomes and effectiveness of new and established health care technologies is a necessary element of evaluation and monitoring strategies.
- The computer-based patient record, which will become a necessary and integral part of health care, is fundamental for monitoring strategies.
- Technology evaluations and decisions should not, in general, be dominated by a preoccupation with the characteristics and demands of individual technologies but rather should derive from the clinical, financial, institutional, and social objectives and needs of those who may benefit or suffer from the technologies.

Committee and staff reviewed the literature on telemedicine, making use of computer-based information resources sponsored by the NLM and other organizations. Although the committee recognized a number of interesting telemedicine initiatives in other countries, it concentrated its limited time and resources on the United States.[2] Committee members and staff participated in site visits, conference calls, and meetings with a variety of individuals and groups. A six-member technical advisory panel (see p. iv) met with

---

[1]The committee drew on a variety of studies that elaborate on many of the listed points. They include IOM reports on health services research (1979, 1995a), computer-based patient records (1991), technology assessment and effectiveness research (1985, 1990a), clinical research (1990b, 1994a), health data systems (1994b), quality assessment and improvement (1989, 1990c), and clinical practice guidelines (1992b). Other agencies have likewise produced important reports on these topics (see, e.g., Shortell and Reinhardt, 1992; OTA, 1986a, 1994, 1995; PPRC, 1989, 1995).

[2]Staff created an inventory of telemedicine projects and evaluations, but the committee concluded that the documentation of completed and ongoing projects was so uneven that the inventory, although useful for the committee, should not be published with the report. In addition, various government agencies were moving through surveys and other means to develop inventories and make them available electronically (Puskin et al., 1995).

the study committee in November 1995 to assist it in defining key evaluation questions and criteria and to provide written comments on preliminary materials drafted by the committee. Committee members prepared background papers on economic and behavioral issues, and these have been incorporated into various sections of this report. The committee reviewed a draft manuscript and discussed final conclusions and recommendations at its third and final meeting in February 1996. This document, which was submitted for outside review in accordance with IOM and National Research Council procedures and policies, constitutes the committee's formal report.

TERMS AND DEFINITIONS

As more and more people use computers and advanced telecommunications technologies at work and at home, the arcane language of these technologies—bits and bytes, analog and digital signals, pixels and bandwidths—is slowly diffusing, but it remains far from common parlance in most medical settings. Reflecting its dependence on these technologies, the field of telemedicine is replete with highly technical terms and abbreviations.

This report tries to avoid jargon when possible and to define clearly those technical terms that are necessary. Because even terms that are in relatively common use may have a variety of explicit— and implicit—definitions, several key terms and concepts are defined and discussed below. Other terms will be defined as they are used in later chapters. A glossary and list of abbreviations are also provided for reference (see Appendix B).

Telemedicine

The committee sought a definition of telemedicine that was parsimonious, consistent with customary social or professional usage, and not easily misunderstood or misused. The group began by reviewing a number of suggested definitions.[3] The common elements of these definitions were (a) information or telecommunica-

---

[3] The definitions consulted by the committee included these:

"the investigation, monitoring and management of patients, and the education of patients and staff using systems which allow ready access to expert advice, no matter where the patient is located" (Van Goord and Christensen, 1992, cited in Gott, 1995, p. 10).

tions technologies, (b) distance between participants, and (c) health or medical uses. The definitions differed in whether they (a) singled out clinical applications or also covered other uses and (b) incorporated the concept of an integrated structure or system. The committee definition incorporates the three common elements. Clinical applications are treated as one category of applications of telemedicine. The committee viewed the degree of system integration not as a defining characteristic but, rather, as a major variable or factor to be considered in planning, implementing, evaluating, and redesigning telemedicine programs to achieve desired outcomes.

Thus, as cited on the first page of this report, *telemedicine* is defined as *the use of electronic information and communications technologies to provide and support health care when distance separates the participants.*[4] Several elements of this definition warrant comment.

"the use of telecommunications techniques at remote sites for the purpose of enhancing diagnoses, expediting research, and improving treatment of illnesses" (Weis, 1993, p. 151).

"the practice of health care delivery, diagnosis, consultation, treatment, transfer of medical data, and education using . . . audio, visual, and data communications" (Kansas Telemedicine Policy Group, 1993, p. 1.6).

"the use of telecommunications technology as a medium for providing health care services for persons that are at some distance from the provider" (Grigsby et al., 1993, p. 1.3).

"the use of two-way, interactive telecommunications video systems to examine patients from remote locations, to facilitate medical consultations, and to train health care professionals" (Council on Competitiveness, 1994, p. 6).

"the use of telecommunications technologies to provide medical information and services" (Perednia and Allen, 1995, p. 483).

"an integrated system of healthcare [sic] delivery and education that employs telecommunications and computer technology as a substitute for face-to-face contact between provider and client" (Bashshur, 1995, p. 19).

"the use of information technology to deliver medical services and information from one location to another" (OTA, 1995, p. 224).

"an infrastructure for furnishing an array of individual services that are performed using telecommunications technologies" (PPRC, 1995, p. 135).

"telemedicine encompasses all of the health care, education, information and administrative services that can be transmitted over distances by telecommunications technologies" (Lipson and Henderson, 1995, p. I-1-4).

"the use of modern telecommunications and information technologies for the provision of clinical care to individuals at a distance and the transmission of information to provide that care" (Puskin, et al., 1995, p. 394).

[4]Derivative terms include: teleconferencing, teleconsultation, telementoring, telepresence, and telemonitoring as well as terms related to specific clinical fields such as teleradiology, teledermatology, and telepsychiatry. The first five terms are defined in the glossary (Appendix B).

First, the committee recognized that video conferencing is sometimes perceived as the defining mode of telemedicine, but the committee's definition more broadly encompasses telephone conversations, transmission of still images, and other communications as well. Further, although the means of transferring information from one location to another (i.e., telecommunications media) are important, they are only a part of the technological base of telemedicine. More generally, information technologies include computer-based means for capturing, storing, manipulating, analyzing, retrieving, and displaying data.

Second, the committee's definition covers both clinical and nonclinical applications of telemedicine. As shown in Table 1.1, current uses fall into several broad categories. *Clinical* applications of telemedicine, the focus of this report, involve the first category—patient care, including diagnostic, treatment, and other medical decisions or services for particular patients. *Nonclinical* uses of telemedicine, such as continuing medical education and management meetings, do not involve decisions about care for specific patients. The clinical-nonclinical boundary is *not* sharp, however. In particular, a primary care physician who views or participates in consultations for a series of similar patients may in the process learn how to diagnose or manage a clinical problem without consultation in most subsequent cases. (To the extent that such learning is one explicit objective of the consultation, the label "telementoring" may be applied.) Moreover, nonclinical uses of telemedicine for administrative or educational purposes may contribute to the effectiveness of clinical applications by encouraging greater familiarity and acceptance of sophisticated telecommunications technologies and by spreading certain capital and operating costs over a larger base.

Third, geographic separation or distance between the participants is a defining characteristic of telemedicine. (The term *distance medicine* is sometimes used as a synonym for telemedicine.) Although many of the technologies employed in telemedicine (e.g., computers) are also used when distance is not an obvious issue (e.g., within a radiology department), telemedicine came into being to overcome problems arising from geographic separation between people who need health care and those who could provide or support an important element of that care.

TABLE 1.1 Categories and Examples of Telemedicine Applications

Category	Examples
Patient care	Radiology consultations; postsurgical monitoring; triage of emergency patients
Professional education	Continuing medical education programs; on-line information and education resources; individual mentoring and instruction
Patient education	On-line help services for patients with chronic health problems
Research	Aggregation of data from multiple sites; conducting and coordinating research at multiple sites
Public health	Access to care for disadvantaged groups; poison control centers; disease reporting
Health care administration	Video conferences for managers of integrated health systems; utilization and quality monitoring

Classifying Clinical Applications of Telemedicine

As noted above, clinical applications of telemedicine involve care for particular individuals, although any given transaction may also serve educational, administrative, or research purposes. In a report that considered telemedicine in the context of provider payment policies, Grigsby et al. (1994a) proposed a broad classification scheme for these applications (see also PPRC, 1995).[5] The commit-

---

[5]The nine categories in this classification covered: (1) initial urgent evaluation of patients; triage decisions; pretransfer arrangements; (2) medical and surgical follow-up, including medication checks; (3) supervision and consultation for primary care encounters in sites where a physician is not available; (4) routine consultations and second opinions based on history, physical exam findings, and available test data; (5) transmission of diagnostic images; (6) extended diagnostic workups or short-term management of self-limited conditions; (7) management of chronic disease and conditions requiring a specialist not available locally; (8) transmission of medical data; and (9) public health, preventive medicine, and patient education.

tee slightly revised this classification by aggregating similar applications to produce six general categories:

1. initial urgent evaluation of patients for triage, stabilization, and transfer decisions;
2. supervision of primary care by nonphysician providers when a physician is not available locally;
3. one-time or continuing provision of specialty care when a specialist is not available locally;
4. consultation, including second opinions;
5. monitoring and tracking of patient status as part of follow-up care or management of chronic problems; and
6. use of remote information and decision analysis resources to support or guide care for specific patients.

This classification scheme includes a mix of several different dimensions related to the clinical problem, the process of care, and the kind of clinical information involved in a particular clinical application of telemedicine. Each of these dimensions, in turn, involves several possible subdimensions, as depicted in Table 1.2.

In this report, the site that organizes and provides telemedicine services is called the *central* or *consulting* site and the site at which the patient is located or from which patient data are initially sent is called the *remote, satellite,* or *distant* site. Those at the central site are often specialist physicians but they may also be primary care physicians, nurse practitioners, psychologists, nutritionists, and other personnel.

Evaluation

Evaluation is a broad term applied to a variety of methods and strategies for identifying the effects and assessing the value, feasibility, or other qualities of a technology, program, or policy. In developing an *evaluation framework*, the committee construed its task as delineating the basic concepts of evaluation and relating them to the particular issues raised by telemedicine.

Evaluations may compare particular clinical interventions (e.g., psychotherapy versus drug treatment for mental disorders) or the programs or systems organized to provide health care services (e.g., inpatient versus outpatient mental health care). Evaluations may

TABLE 1.2 Dimensions, Subdimensions, and Examples of Patient Care Relevant to Telemedicine Applications

Dimension	Subdimension and Examples
Clinical problems	Urgency, complexity, pathophysiology, and persistence. Applications may vary depending on whether they involve • emergency or urgent problems for which prompt evaluation and management is important; • acute problems that may be evaluated and treated on a scheduled basis and that have generally predictable periods of resolution following treatment; • chronic problems that require monitoring and management over a long time period.
Processes of care	Type of care, source of care, source of clinical information. Applications may vary depending on whether they involve • prevention, diagnosis, treatment, rehabilitation, or monitoring; • generalist care or specialty care; • remote-site clinicians, patients, or technical personnel; • interactive examination or questioning of a patient (or patient data) or deferred use of recorded information.
Clinical information	Aural, visual, numerical, textual.[a] Applications may vary depending on whether they involve • sounds (e.g., speech, chest sounds); • pictures (e.g., still photos, full-motion video, radiologic images); • graphic data (e.g., electrocardiograms); or • alpha-numeric text (e.g., patient history, lab results, practice guidelines).

[a]Of the five major kinds of sensory data (sight, sound, touch, smell, taste), telemedicine routinely transmits only the first two, but these two provide most of the core sensory information for clinical decisionmaking. The transmission of tactile data, which is important for many diagnostic, management, and treatment purposes, is largely experimental (e.g., the "virtual glove" that would allow remote palpation of patients); and the transmission (not just the description) of odors and flavors is, for now, largely unexplored.

focus on processes or outcomes or both. The outcomes of interest may be relatively restricted (e.g., safety but not effectiveness or costs) or a wide range of outcomes may be examined. Evaluations of *efficacy* such as randomized clinical trials test interventions under strictly controlled conditions to minimize the impact of "extraneous" variables, whereas evaluations of *effectiveness* attempt to test interventions under ordinary conditions and to identify how such extraneous variables affect results (Brook and Lohr, 1985).

For purposes of this report, an *evaluation criterion* is a measure, indicator, standard, or similar basis for describing outcomes or making judgments. Examples of criteria in common use in evaluations include mortality, hospital length of stay, and patient satisfaction. The committee focused on the set of basic concerns about the quality, accessibility, and cost of health care that lie at the core of most health services research and technology assessments. Because a comprehensive presentation of specific criteria appropriate for the heterogeneity of telemedicine applications was beyond the committee's resources, this report sets forth criteria in the form of questions with examples of the kinds of measures or standards that would be applied to particular telemedicine applications.

Drawing from a widely cited 1990 IOM report, the committee agreed that *quality* of care is "the degree to which health care services for individuals and populations increase the likelihood of desired health outcomes and are consistent with current professional knowledge" (IOM 1990c, p. 21). Consistent with the concepts set forth in a 1993 report (IOM, 1993a), the committee defined *access* as the timely receipt of appropriate health care. *Costs* measure the value of resources expended for an activity or objective. They are generally measured in dollars but are sometimes expressed in other units (e.g., travel time, days lost from work, treatment delays) without monetary conversion. These concepts and related evaluation topics (e.g., cost-effectiveness) are discussed further in later chapters of this report.

Although many telemedicine evaluations will focus on individual patient care, the growth of managed care and the debate over allocating resources for health care will direct more evaluations toward populations, including but not limited to those enrolled in managed care plans. Analyses may compare the costs, benefits, and risks of alternative services for an entire population or may concentrate on outcomes for the least healthy or most vulnerable groups in a population (e.g., elderly individuals, teenage mothers). For example, a telemedicine application might target a high-risk group to test whether telemonitoring, on-line information services, and early intervention could reduce total medical costs compared to conventional care.

STRUCTURE OF THE REPORT

This chapter has described the origins of this project and presented principles and definitions on which the remaining chapters build. The rest of this report provides a broad context and framework for evaluations that would expand information for decisionmakers considering telemedicine.

The next four chapters provide context. Chapter 2 reviews the evolution of telemedicine and illustrates the range of current applications. Chapter 3 considers the technical and human infrastructure of telemedicine, and Chapter 4 discusses policy issues with an emphasis on professional licensure, malpractice, medical privacy, payment for services, and telecommunications law. Chapter 5 reviews telemedicine evaluation frameworks and selected evaluation projects identified by the committee. As noted earlier, the focus is on programs in the United States.

The committee sets forth basic principles of evaluation and proposes elements for telemedicine evaluation in Chapter 6. Chapter 7 is organized around the quality, access, and cost outcomes but also considers patient and provider acceptance of telemedicine. The report concludes in Chapter 8 with the committee's findings and recommendations.

One theme runs through this report. Although telemedicine involves a large and quite varied assortment of clinical practices, devices, and organizational arrangements, its applications should be subject conceptually to the same evaluation principles as apply (or should apply) to other technologies in health care.

2

Evolution and Current Applications of Telemedicine

EVOLUTION OF DISTANCE COMMUNICATION

People have been communicating over considerable distances by sounds or visible signals for centuries. Drums, horns, and other instruments have been used—and are still used in some places—to send messages using certain sound patterns that correspond to prearranged codes. In one of the greatest of the Greek tragedies, *Agamemnon*, Aeschylus begins his drama with word of beacon fires carrying news of the fall of Troy and the return of the king—news that set in motion Clytemnestra's plan to kill her husband in long-delayed revenge for his slaying of their daughter. These signal fires would have required a series of line-of-site beacons stretching 500 miles across the Aegean Sea (Encyclopedia Britannica, 1989). Today, some 2,500 years after Aeschylus and 3,000 years after the events of the legend, line-of-sight transmission remains important as a critical element of modern microwave relay systems.

Not until the 1700s and 1800s, however, did a series of electrical inventions make possible a subsequent, dramatic expansion in the availability of near-instantaneous communication across long distances. This expansion began in the United States with the inauguration of intercity public telegraph services between Washington and Baltimore in 1844. During the Civil War, the military ordered medical supplies and transmitted casualty lists by telegraph, and it seems probable that some uses of the telegraph in its early decades involved medical consultations (Zundel, 1996).

In 1876, Alexander Graham Bell patented the telephone, a device for electronic speech transmission. Bell's investigations arose, in part, from experiments to develop multiplex telegraphy that would allow several telegraph messages to be sent simultaneously over the same wire.

Commercial applications quickly followed Bell's patent, and long-distance telephone links began to appear in the 1880s. Since then, a continuing stream of technological innovations has improved the usefulness of telephone communication. These innovations include manual switchboards to connect multiple telephone lines, loaded circuits to reduce distortion over long distances, vacuum tube amplifiers to boost signals, and automatic switching systems, to name just a few. Telephone circuits can also carry still and video images as well as audio signals and data, and radio signals have been used to extend the reach of telephone communication.

These technical advances significantly extended the foundation on which telemedicine could build. Furthermore, at least five generations of users have created and passed on a legacy of technologies, behaviors, and expectations that make telephone communication commonplace. Parents give children telephone toys and let them answer real telephones at an early age; adults who find a child answering their calls generally tolerate and even enjoy participating in this early education in telephone technology. The other technologies on which telemedicine relies, such as the personal computer work station, are at varying stages of integration into everyday personal life or health care delivery.

As context for the committee's evaluation framework, this chapter briefly reviews the development of telemedicine and provides examples of current clinical applications. Chapter 3 provides more background on the technical and human infrastructure that supports telemedicine.

DEVELOPMENT OF TELEMEDICINE

In April 1924, an imaginative cover for the magazine *Radio*

News foreshadowed telemedicine in its depiction of a "radio doctor" linked to a patient not only by sound but also by a live picture (Figure 2.1). At the time, radio had just begun to reach into American homes, and the first experimental television transmission did not actually occur until 1927. (See Figure 2.3 for a 1990s image of telemedicine.)

The magazine cover also illustrates the attention-getting character of interactive video applications in telemedicine. Ordinary telephone calls to the doctor's office and even 911 calls are so commonplace today that they are often overlooked and rarely evaluated as telemedicine applications. Nonetheless, in many situations, they are the alternative to which more complex clinical uses of telemedicine should be compared. Similarly, when visual information is an essential part of a consultation, the relevant options include still as well as moving images, and both kinds of images can be sent and received on a delayed rather than real-time base. With the telephone, such delay is common and accepted, for example, when a nurse says "I'll give this information to the doctor and we'll get back to you later today" or when a physician promises to call about test results.

According to one review, the first reference to telemedicine in the medical literature appeared in 1950 (Zundel, 1996). The article described the transmission, beginning in 1948, of radiologic images by telephone between West Chester and Philadelphia, Pennsylvania, a distance of 24 miles (Gershon-Cohen and Cooley, 1950). Building on this early work, Canadian radiologists at Montreal's Jean-Talon Hospital created a teleradiology system in the 1950s (Allen, 1996; Allen and Allen, 1994b).

Medical uses of video communications in the United States are commonly dated to 1959 (see, e.g., Bashshur et al., 1975; Perednia and Allen, 1995). In that year, clinicians at the University of Nebraska used two-way interactive television to transmit neurological examinations and other information across campus to medical students (Benschoter et al., 1967; Wittson and Benschoter, 1972). They next explored its use for group therapy consultations, and in 1964 they established a telemedicine link with the Norfolk State Hospital (112 miles away) to provide speech therapy, neurological examinations, diagnosis of difficult psychiatric cases, case consultations, research seminars, and education and training.

Also in 1959, a Canadian radiologist reported diagnostic consul-

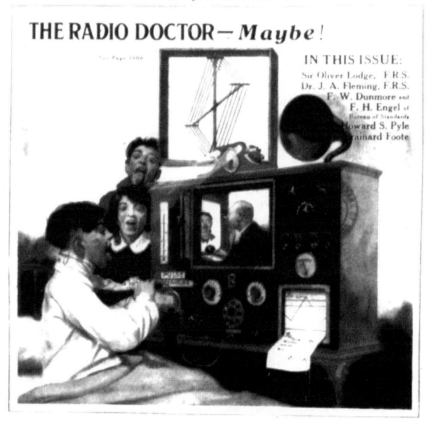

FIGURE 2.1　Telemedicine circa 1924—visionary cover of *Radio News* depicting an imagined "radio doctor" who could see and be seen by his patient. The first experimental television transmission did not occur until 1927. Photo courtesy of the Radiology Information System Consortium, Reston, Virginia.

tations based on fluoroscopy images transmitted by coaxial cable (Jutra, 1959). In 1961, the journal *Anesthesiology* reported on radiotelemetry for patient monitoring (Davis et al., 1961). Ship-to-shore transmission of electrocardiograms (ECGs) and x-rays was reported in 1965 (Monnier et al., 1965),[1] and transoceanic transmission was reported soon thereafter (Hirschman et al., 1967).

Although the Nebraska program and many of the other early telemedicine applications arose out of concerns about the limited access of remote populations to a variety of health services, urban uses also appeared fairly early. In 1967, physicians at the University of Miami School of Medicine and the City of Miami Fire Department reported their pioneering use of existing voice radio channels to transmit electrocardiographic rhythms from fire-rescue units to Jackson Memorial Hospital (Nagel et al., 1968). Today, it is commonplace for paramedics to transmit cardiac rhythms and 12-lead ECGs to hospital emergency departments. These and certain other kinds of emergency telemetry are now so routine and so much a part of mainstream health care that they are often not mentioned as telemedicine applications.

In another early use of telecommunications technologies to assist in urban emergency and urgent situations, Massachusetts General Hospital (MGH) established in 1963 a telecommunications link with a medical station staffed by nurse clinicians at Boston's Logan Airport (Bird, 1972). In 1968, MGH added an interactive television microwave link that provided electrocardiograph, stethoscope, microscopy, voice, and other capabilities. During the same period, MGH also established a telepsychiatry link with the Veterans Administration Hospital in Bedford, Massachusetts, that continued to operate until the mid-1980s (Crump and Pfeil, 1995).

A report from the National Academy of Engineering (NAE) on communications technologies in urban areas suggested other uses of telemedicine that would be applicable in urban as well as rural areas (NAE, 1971). One such use involved physician services for nursing home patients; another use involved the supervision of nonphysician providers in ambulatory care clinics. The Mt. Sinai School of Medicine in New York City tested the latter application when it established in 1972 a black-and-white cable television link to support

---

[1]This 1965 article dated the first telephone transmission of electrocardiograms to 1906.

nurse practitioners providing pediatric primary care at a clinic in an Hispanic area of the city (Muller et al., 1977).

In the 1960s and 1970s, various other telemedicine applications were initiated, several of which were supported by federal agencies including the U.S. Department of Health, Education and Welfare (what is now the Department of Health and Human Services, DHHS) and the National Aeronautics and Space Administration (NASA). An unusual set of partners—the U.S. Indian Health Service, NASA, and the Lockheed Company—joined in sponsoring STARPAHC (Space Technology Applied to Rural Papago[2] Advanced Health Care), which tested satellite-based communications to provide medical services to astronauts and to residents of an isolated reservation. The STARPAHC project lasted for about 20 years with most of its elements being phased out in the late 1970s.

In addition, the U.S. Public Health Service and the Department of Defense sponsored a series of teleradiology projects in the 1970s and 1980s (Gayler et al., 1979; Gitlin, 1986). These projects led to the collaborative Digital Imaging Network Project to promote the development and implementation of civilian and military teleradiology (Greberman et al., 1988; Mun et al., 1989). In the 1980s, some radiologists began to use inexpensive systems for "on-call" screening of images (Gitlin, 1994).

According to Perednia and Allen (1995), only one of the formal telemedicine programs that was started before 1986 survived into the mid-1990s. That program, established by the Memorial University of Newfoundland, began in 1977 with a three-month demonstration project involving one-way television and two-way audio. The test was "successful" in demonstrating the value of television, but the project team concluded that much of the educational material and data could be provided efficiently and less expensively by telephone, videotape, audio teleconferencing, and print materials (House, 1993).[3] The university is still using telemedicine to support

---

[2]The name now used for this tribe is Tohono O'odham.

[3]These findings are consistent with those reported in 1977 by Dunn et al. In a study that compared on-site physician diagnoses with remote physician diagnoses using telephone, still-frame black-and-white television, black-and-white television, and color television, few differences were found among the options. This led the authors to "question the advisability of building expensive broad-band video systems to assist in the delivery of primary health care . . . [when the alternatives] are substantially cheaper, generally more reliable, and appear to provide equally effective health care management (Dunn et al., 1977, p. 29).

a range of clinical, educational, and research activities, most of which are not video based.

Also illustrating the fluctuating interest in telemedicine in the past, a 1992 literature review found that the National Library of Medicine information system included 127 articles on health care uses of telemedicine and 55 articles on educational uses for the period 1975–1982 whereas the 1983–1990 period showed only 75 articles in the former area and 117 in the latter (Crump and Pfeil, 1995). The authors of this review cite high transmission costs as a major reason for the waning of interest in telemedicine in the early and mid-1980s. They note that improved technologies and lower costs began to revive interest in telemedicine toward the end of the 1980s. More recent literature searches reflect this renewed interest (Scannell et al., 1995).

CURRENT APPLICATIONS OF TELEMEDICINE

Growth and Diversity

The number of telemedicine users is now expanding rapidly enough that no complete inventory of applications is available, especially for projects involving private nonprofit and commercial sponsorship or funding. To fill that information gap, a federal working group on telemedicine (discussed further in Chapters 4 and 5) is developing an inventory that will initially include government projects and then expand to include state and private projects (Puskin et al., 1995). Part of that effort has included a survey to identify rural hospitals using telemedicine in one form or another. The Department of Defense and the Department of Veterans Affairs are likewise working to document more fully telemedicine activities at their facilities. Private organizations have also been tracking and reporting public and private telemedicine programs (Telemedicine Monitor, 1995). For example, the state health policy program of George Washington University surveyed and analyzed state government initiatives to support telemedicine as discussed further in Chapter 4 (Lipson and Henderson, 1995).

Most tracking efforts focus on programs transmitting still images (e.g., radiologic images) or using interactive television. One recent overview estimated that the number of programs using the latter technology has reached 50, with growth doubling each year between 1990 and 1995 (Allen and Perednia, 1996). The review also suggested that teleradiology installations were growing at a similar pace, although getting accurate data on these programs has not been easy, in part because vendors have been reluctant to release sales information (Franken, 1996).

Newspapers, medical newsletters, and other sources document the development of the Internet as a vehicle for the formal and informal provision of medical advice. An increasing number of health-related organizations are establishing World Wide Web pages (including a number of programs described in this report),[4] and a variety of individuals and groups have created less formal "chat groups" and other links that respond to many consumers for greater self-determination in medical care.[5]

The diversity of telemedicine demonstration projects is suggested by the 19 projects funded by the Office of Rural Health Policy (see Appendix A). The discussion below, which includes some of these projects, further illustrates the range of clinical applications of telemedicine. It includes both common and relatively uncommon applications. Some examples focus on clinical specialties (e.g., radiology) whereas others focus on populations or sites of care (e.g., prisons). Most programs have received governmental grants or other public subsidies, but some are essentially self-sustaining. This diversity underscores the challenge of designing evaluation strategies, measures, and data collection methods to fit different settings, populations, clinical conditions, and objectives.

Teleradiology

As indicated earlier, the most common current applications of telemedicine (other than general telephone and fax communications) appear to involve radiologic image transmission within and among

---

[4]Health information sources on the World Wide Web can be searched using a variety of "search engines" such as Yahoo (http://www.yahoo.com/Health/) and EINet (http://einet.net/galaxy/Medicine.html) and other sources such as the Telemedicine Information Exchange (http://tie.telemed.org) and Medical Matrix (http://www.slackinc.com/matrix). The latter site is sponsored by the American Medical Informatics Association's Internet Working Group.

[5]One committee member cited a chat-group participant from Taiwan who described a relative with an illness the local doctors had not diagnosed; suggestions made by other participants assisted the subsequent local diagnosis (John Scott, personal communication, February 6, 1995).

health care organizations. Several steps are typically involved in teleradiology including digitizing film images or directly producing digital images, incorporating demographic and other patient information, compressing images (data) in various ways to allow them to be sent more quickly and inexpensively, transmitting images from one site to another, and reconstructing images for viewing and interpretation (Forsberg, 1995). Additional steps are required for storing and retrieving images electronically.

The growth of teleradiology applications reflects several characteristics of radiology: (a) its well-established consulting infrastructure based on mail and courier services; (b) its early use of digital imaging technologies; and (c) the availability of Medicare payment for teleradiology consultations. Radiology centers have long used mailed or courier-delivered films to provide, as described by one organization, "consultation, second opinions, and primary interpretations; image over-read [and other educational and supportive services] for individuals getting started in MR [magnetic resonance imaging] or other difficult modalities; quality control of image interpretation; vacation coverage; and additional coverage for groups with an increasing case volume as yet insufficient to justify hiring an additional radiologist" (UCSF, 1995). In many situations, teleradiology can make such distance services much quicker and more convenient, and the electronic storage of images minimizes problems with mislaid or lost films as images move between or within organizations. Radiologists can also have images transmitted to home or office work stations so they may not have to go to the hospital to see films when they are on call.

A second base for teleradiology is the relatively early experience in radiology with the advantages and complexities of computer-based digital technologies such as computed axial tomography and magnetic resonance imaging. These were followed by other technologies such as picture archiving and communication systems and advanced digital switching, which provided the option of high-quality electronic transmission of images. These developments made institutional adoption of digital radiology feasible and facilitated the development of multi-institutional teleradiology networks. Several sites on the World Wide Web provide radiology and pathology images for educational purposes, and some programs are testing or using pathology and radiology transmission for clinical purposes (Hancock, 1995; Allen and Perednia, 1996).

Particularly critical for teleradiology is a third element: Medicare and other coverage policies that have allowed payment for radiology consultations without the face-to-face interaction required for most other consultations. This requirement is a major source of frustration for many advocates of other telemedicine applications.[6] (See Chapter 4 for further discussion of payment issues.)

Most teleradiology applications have built on conventional film-based radiology programs. To cite one example, the University of Iowa began in 1987 to add teleradiology to an established film-based radiology program (Franken, 1996). The university now provides a variety of teleradiology services to rural sites within the state. In one experimental program, the university uses teleradiology to provide 80 percent of the coverage to a 30-bed rural hospital.

For the Veterans Affairs (VA) Medical Center in Baltimore, Maryland, teleradiology was an outgrowth of a more fundamental decision to adopt (except for mammography) a filmless or digital radiology technology throughout the new facility being built in the early 1990s (Siegel, 1996). The center has both a commercial picture archiving and communication system (PACS) and a system that is part of the VA's Decentralized Hospital Computer Program, which acquires, stores, and displays images and other information from other departments. From this base, the Baltimore center has begun providing teleradiology services to four smaller VA facilities in the region. Other VA facilities are developing teleradiology based on conventional and filmless systems.

In general, the wider use of digital radiology within health care centers can be expected to provide an additional impetus for tele-

---

[6]For instance, teledermatology is not yet widespread, although dermatological problems are a common source of requests for consultations in telemedicine programs. In its test of telemedicine to support deployed troops in Somalia and elsewhere, the military has found a high frequency of dermatology consults (Walters, 1996). Similarly, reports on prison telemedicine programs indicate a high proportion of such consults (Allen, 1995a). In both military and prison settings, payer concerns about overutilization of services are less acute than in fee-for-service arrangements. The availability of research documenting the quality and cost-effectiveness of teledermatology could make it attractive to managed care organizations, in which financial and other incentives make overuse of consultations less of a concern.

radiology to expand beyond institutional boundaries. Multi-institutional teleradiology networks are emerging. Telequest, for example, is a teleradiology venture recently created by five academic medical centers (Bowman Gray, the Brigham and Women's Hospital, Emory University, the University of California at San Francisco, and the University of Pennsylvania) (Gore, 1996). Some of the individual and multi-institutional teleradiology ventures are probably outgrowths, in part, of excess medical center capacity in the United States (see Pew Health Professions Commission, 1995; IOM, 1996). They illustrate how academic medical centers may look to telemedicine as a way to expand markets nationally and internationally and to offset revenue losses in a changing health care and government environment. As two experienced academic teleradiology experts have described it, "to be digitally aware is to realize the new era of competition" in a cost-constrained environment (Mun and Freedman, 1996).

One additional argument for teleradiology is that it has the potential to improve the quality and reduce the variability of image interpretation. This long-standing concern in the field arises because general radiologists may spend only a small portion of their time on certain tasks such as mammogram interpretation and may lack the knowledge and volume of experience of subspecialists (Beam et al., 1996). On the other hand, debate continues about the diagnostic accuracy of teleradiology, quality assurance requirements, and the appropriate trade-offs between accuracy and more timely consultation in some areas (Forsberg, 1995; Franken, 1996). A number of studies have compared digital or digitized images and film (see Chapter 5), but the broader quality implications of teleradiology have yet to be evaluated.

Care in the Home and Other Nonclinical Sites

The use of telemedicine in home and other nonclinical settings illustrates the significance of nonvideo means for providing information and advice and for monitoring patient status. The most familiar nonvideo telemedicine option is the use of the telephone. Physicians, nurses, and other personnel routinely talk with patients and families—providing information, checking their status, and offering reassurance—without the expense or inconvenience of an office visit for the patient or a home visit for the clinician. To reduce avoidable office visits, many health plans have established telephone advisory programs, staffed primarily by nurses, to provide patients with information, assessments, and recommendations for routine medical problems. For medical and other emergencies, the 911 system works from any telephone to put people in touch with dispatchers who assess the nature of the emergency, send medical or other assistance as indicated, and provide medical instructions (e.g., for cardiopulmonary resuscitation) when necessary.

In addition to person-to-person communications, automated telephone services are used in various ways. For example, interactive voice response systems allow individuals to initiate calls and respond to recorded questions using a touch-tone telephone. Such systems have been used to test automated telephone screening for depression, with questionnaire scores provided to callers along with toll-free follow-up telephone numbers (Baer et al., 1995). A different kind of automated arrangement provides for scheduled, automatic calls to patients. Patients can then respond by using a touch-tone telephone to enter basic medical information or by using a special device attached to the telephone to transmit physiological measurements. Evaluations of these kinds of program are discussed in Chapter 5.

One of the oldest telephone-based monitoring programs has been operated by Veterans Affairs Medical Centers in San Francisco and Washington, D.C. They have acted as pacemaker surveillance centers since 1982, and these centers now monitor over 11,000 patients both at home and away from home (VA, 1996). (Because pacemakers are programmed to change their normal operating frequency when batteries run low and because an electrocardiogram can detect this problem, a device attached to a telephone can transfer an ECG reading to the centers, which can thus identify this problem long distance.) Other monitoring systems rely on radio-based technologies to raise an alarm if a patient does not check in on a regular basis or if a patient triggers the alarm following an emergency such as a fall. Patients with heart disease can carry beepers that allow them—if they experience symptoms—to transmit a 12-lead electrocardiogram using ordinary phone lines. A commercial service in Israel claims 30,000 subscribers for such a system (Carthy, 1995).

Video-based home health options are also varied but less common. Many are still in the testing stage. Patients may sit before video cameras at scheduled times to talk with clinicians and, perhaps, display skin conditions, demonstrate their range of motion, show thermometer readings, or otherwise offer visual information about their condition. A variety of instruments may also be attached to home video units to transmit heart sounds, blood pressure measurements, and other patient data. The term "electronic housecall" is an attention-getting description often applied to such combinations of video and other technologies for home monitoring and consultation (Jones, 1993).

Finally, no discussion of home-based telemedicine can ignore the growth of Internet services, which offer a wide range of general information and other services that can be used in many settings (Johannes, 1996; Lamberg, 1996; Borzo, 1996b). A quick search of the World Wide Web will turn up a myriad of general and specialized information sites on dozens of health issues, some aimed at patients, others at clinicians (see footnote 3 above). In addition, groups of people with common health problems ranging from minor to severe can share information and concerns through a variety of Internet services. Electronic mail also provides an alternative to telephone conversations between clinician and patient, clinician and clinician, and patient and patient. The extent to which the Internet may overtake other telemedicine transmission arrangements for a variety of hospital and clinic settings is a subject of considerable debate.

Telemedicine for Prison Populations

State officials are showing increasing interest in the potential of telemedicine to provide better access for prisoners to timely generalist and specialist consultations and to reduce the costs and inconvenience associated with current on-site and off-site arrangements (Allen, 1995a,b; Braly, 1995; Lipson and Henderson, 1995; Brecht et al., 1996; Chinnock, 1996). Colorado, North Carolina, and Texas are among the states with operational programs, and other states are considering or testing programs. A major objective of prison telemedicine is to avoid the high costs of either bringing medical specialists to prison (the costs of which are high partially owing to adverse working conditions) or transporting the patient (the costs of which are high because at least two guards and a state vehicle are required for security). In North Carolina, it is estimated that the average prisoner transport cost for medical services is over $700 (Kesler and

Balch, 1995). In addition, prisoner programs also are expected to reduce public concern about prisoner escapes, provide earlier access to care and better access to subspecialty care, and supply videotaped documentation of services that may be useful in lawsuits. Because prison telemedicine programs are generating relatively large number of cases, they offer considerable potential for systematic evaluation such as those undertaken and planned by Texas Tech and the University of Texas Medical Branch at Galveston.

One early program has been operated by the East Carolina University (ECU) School of Medicine, which is also involved in other telemedicine projects that are linked to a statewide distance learning network established in 1989 (Kesler and Balch, 1995; OTA, 1995; Keppler, 1996; Tichenor et al., 1996). ECU provides telemedicine services to the maximum security Central Prison, which has two physicians working at the facility 100 miles distant in Raleigh, North Carolina. The program began in 1992, prompted by a combination of an increasing prison population and legal challenges focused on prisoners' right to health care. The initial focus was emergency consultations between the prison health unit and the emergency department at the University Medical Center. The program now includes 31 ECU physicians from 15 medical disciplines.[7] A financial audit of the North Carolina Department of Corrections in March 1994 found evidence of cost savings by the Central Prison Telemedicine Project, but this analysis has not been published. The audit did, however, lead to a formal recommendation that the program be extended to more prison facilities around the state. The quality of care has not been formally evaluated.

Rural Telepsychiatry

One of the nonradiology programs that has moved beyond demonstration status is RODEO NET (Rural Options for Development and Educational Opportunities). It began in 1988 when community mental health programs in 13 eastern Oregon counties organized the Eastern Oregon Human Services Consortium (EOHSC). In 1991,

---

[7]At the time of last checking (June 1996) on the Web page for the entire ECU program (http://150.216.193.51/r-folder/consult.html), 890 consultations had been performed, over half (495) of which involved dermatology. Other frequently consulted specialties include neurology (85) and gastroenterology (94).

EOHSC was awarded a three-year ($700,000) grant from the Office of Rural Health Policy (ORHP) to demonstrate the use of telecommunications in delivering mental health care in eastern Oregon, a large rural area remote from many secondary and tertiary medical resources (ORHP, 1993b; Allen and Allen, 1994a). Operations began in 1992 and the project has since become independent of federal grant funding (Britain, 1995; OTA, 1995).

On the clinical side, the telepsychiatry program is used for case consultation (both one-time and ongoing), patient evaluation, medication management, and crisis response through a 24-hour psychiatric emergency service. Administrative, educational, and other uses include preadmission, predischarge, and transfer reviews; precommitment and recommitment hearings; continuing health professions education; technology training for both consumers and providers; peer networking; and management video conferencing. Available interactive services include a one-way video, a two-way audio, and a two-way compressed video/audio/data link.

Current funding sources include service contracts with EOHSC, Greater Oregon Behavioral Health, Inc. (a nonprofit managed behavioral health care organization responsible for delivering public behavioral health care services to consumers in eastern Oregon under the Oregon Health Plan demonstration), and Oregon's Mental Health and Developmental Disability Services Division. A public-private partnership consisting of Greater Oregon Behavioral Health, Inc., Oregon ED-NET (a public telecommunication service providing satellite video conferencing), and Eastern Oregon State College helped fund some of the program's technical infrastructure. Rural sites lease equipment from Oregon ED-NET and pay a $5,000 yearly membership fee in addition to a charge for air time. The network also receives fees for training offered over the system.

In discussing the program's ability to become self-sustaining, the program director cited several factors during video-conference comments to committee members visiting Oregon Health Sciences University (Catherine Britain, November 1995). First, the program arose as a cooperative, grass-roots initiative to solve the clearly recognized problem of limited availability of mental health services for a sparsely populated area. It was viewed as a means of meeting health needs, not as an end in itself. Second, the creation of a public-private partnership increased the base across which telecommunications infrastructure costs could be spread. Third, the program had some key champions who remained committed to the effort in the face of continuing technical, political, administrative, and other problems. Fourth, training and support for users focused on establishing comfort with technologies at a level equivalent to that for the telephone.

Postsurgical Monitoring in an Urban Nursing Home

The postsurgical monitoring program developed by Stanford University Medical Center and nearby Lytton Gardens Health Care Center offers an example of a telemedicine application prompted by local initiative without federal grant funding.[8] This program grew out of discussions initiated by Lytton Gardens, a skilled nursing and residential facility that provides a continuum of services and living arrangements for low-income senior citizens. The Center's Chief Executive Officer (CEO) proposed that telemedicine could be used to assist in the earlier discharge of complicated surgical cases from the medical center to the nursing facility. The first test involved liver transplant patients, followed by reconstructive plastic and vascular surgery patients. The surgeons receive progress notes from the physician and nurses at the nursing facility, and they can examine patients who are brought to a room equipped with a special video camera (operated by a licensed practical nurse) and an audio link that allow both visual inspection of surgical wounds and conversation with the patient. Using the interactive video link, the nursing home has also initiated some psychiatric and dermatology consultations and is considering their use in home care.

Stanford's telemedicine program has received funding for transmission costs from Pacific Bell (a regional Bell operating company recently slated for merger with another regional company) and equipment and software on loan from Hewlett-Packard and md/tv (a medical software company) that will have to be purchased after two years. (Figure 2.2 shows a consultant's telemedicine work station, similar to that used at Stanford. Figure 2.3 shows what a patient might see at a remote site, in this case, a dialysis center.) The postsurgical monitoring program began in June 1995 without imme-

---

[8]This discussion is based primarily on interviews with Christopher Barnard, Medical Director of the Stanford Telemedicine Program and Vera Goupille, Chief Executive Officer of Lytton Gardens and on a brochure, *The Telemedicine Program at Stanford*.

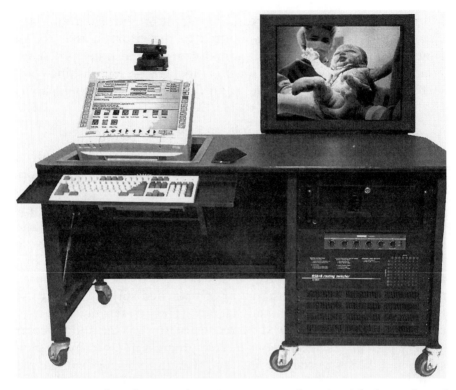

FIGURE 2.2 Telemedicine work station—an example as it might be configured with hardware and software for a consulting clinician to conduct live videoconferencing, capture and transmit images and other data on a store-and-forward basis, share information from the patient record, and perform on-line medical literature searches. The unit includes a personal computer, robotic (pan-tilt-zoom) video camera (mounted above the computer monitor), large video display monitor, microphone, speakers, CODEC (an electronic COder/DECoder device), and software for a variety of purposes including control of some peripheral devices at the remote site. At the remote site, the installation would include a similar set up plus the peripheral devices (e.g., Doppler stethoscope, high-resolution digital still-image camera, full-motion video camera), document scanners, and other equipment appropriate for the patients to be evaluated. Photo used with permission of md/tv, inc., a subsidiary of Multimedia Medical Systems.

diate prospects for insurer payments to either Stanford or Lytton Gardens for the tele-medicine consultations. For Stanford, however, the arrangement provides the benefit of reduced hospital stays, which is financially advantageous since the medical center receives a fixed per-case payment for many of its surgical cases. The CEO of Lytton Gardens sees the benefit of the program in increased referrals from

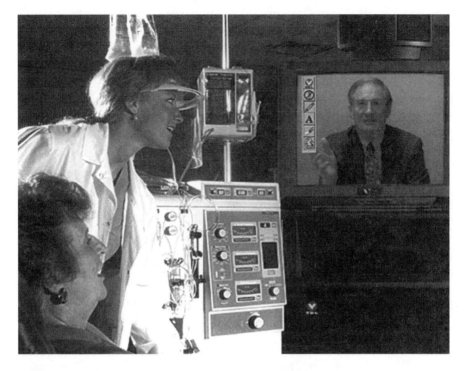

FIGURE 2.3 Telemedicine consultation from the patient's perspective—what a patient (in this case, a patient at a dialyis center) might see during a real-time video consultation with a distant specialist. The patient sees the consultant on one monitor and herself on another (not shown). A robotic video camera is mounted above one of the monitors. Photo used with permission of VTEL.

Stanford, reimbursement at higher levels for more complex patients, and increased satisfaction and retention of nursing staff.

More generally, telemedicine has been factored into strategic business planning for the Stanford University Medical Center, which has made clear that it expects the program to be self-supporting within a few years. One objective is contractual arrangements with HMOs and similar organizations, which are vital in California, a state that is dominated by managed care plans. Stanford already has one such contract with the San Jose Medical Group for dermatology services, and it also is linked to the Drew Health Foundation (a community health center) for telecardiology services, with other services to be added in the future.

Telemedicine in a Managed Care System

As indicated in Chapter 1, the committee found managed care decisionmakers preoccupied with other priorities in health care markets that have become fiercely competitive and increasingly complex politically. Telemedicine did not appear to be a priority, although a few managed care plans are testing clinical and administrative roles for telemedicine. Convincing reports of feasible urban and suburban applications (e.g., for specialist consultations) and cost savings (e.g., from further concentrating specialist services) could spur much greater interest. The expansion of managed care into more rural areas may also spark increased attention.

One integrated health system that is testing telemedicine is Allina, a relatively new, not-for-profit system in Minnesota that resulted from the merger of an insurance company (Medica) and a large health care delivery system (Healthspan) that included a number of rural sites.[9] The organization's telemedicine system has administrative, educational, and community service as well as clinical uses. It is being constructed with a mix of funds including internal resources, a grant from the ORHP, contracts and other arrangements with a consortium of rural hospitals (the Rural Health Alliance), technical assistance from several vendors, and an arrangement with U.S. West (the regional Bell operating company) that lets the system avoid long distance charges for its rural links. The insurance component of Allina pays for telemedicine consultations just as it would pay for any other accepted specialty consultation. The network began operating May 1, 1995, and now serves approximately two dozen urban and rural sites, including the corporate office in Minneapolis. Clinical consultations were initially limited (about 150 from May 1995 to February 1996) but are reported to be growing.

Allina is also testing a link with three very small emergency departments (including two that are not part of the Allina system) located in communities with fewer than 4,000 residents. They are linked with one of Allina's larger rural hospitals, which is staffed 24

---

[9]This discussion is based on committee and staff interviews with Dr. William Goodall of Allina Healthcare Systems and a brochure *Telemedicine: Making the Impossible Possible* put together by Allina and the Rural Health Alliance Telemedicine Network, a consortium of eight rural Minnesota hospitals. See also Cunningham, 1995.

hours a day with certified emergency or family medicine physicians. The central and remote sites can be linked within five minutes. For minor problems, the consulting physician examines the patient through a video/audio link and an on-site nurse carries out orders as appropriate. For more serious cases, additional patient data (e.g., laboratory results, ultrasound, radiographs) may be transmitted so that a decision can be made whether to treat locally or transfer the patient to the larger facility.

The business analysis and strategy behind this arrangement has several elements. The remote sites have been spending up to $70,000 for backup emergency services of uneven quality. Allina could offer them the telemedicine link and transfer arrangement for $40,000 to $50,000 on a contractual basis and could sometimes successfully bill patients' insurers for services. Allina's rural hospital would be expected to increase its emergency care volume and revenues (from both transferred patients and consultations) enough to justify round-the-clock operation. The smaller satellite hospitals would increase their stability and save on the costs of backup emergency care and would likely keep some patients who would otherwise be sent elsewhere.

CONCLUSION

This chapter has briefly reviewed the history of telemedicine and illustrated a range of current applications. The historical review shows an initial emphasis on access objectives for rural areas, with recently increasing interest in urban and suburban uses. Although much attention is paid to interactive video applications, the committee was impressed by the continuing importance of telephone-based and other communications of many kinds.

During its deliberations, the committee heard considerable concern that many current demonstration and other pilot projects would share the fate of most of the 1960s and 1970s projects by not surviving the end of federal grant funding or other subsidies (Cunningham, 1995). Failure to link projects to major organizational plans and business objectives and poor planning were cited as problems. High transmission costs, awkward and quickly outdated technologies, low patient volume, lack of physician interest, and limited insurance coverage also contribute to concerns about program survival.

Chapters 3 and 4 discuss further some of the technical, human, and policy factors that may support or impede the successful introduction and widespread adoption of telemedicine applications such as those described here. If those planning for the implementation and evaluation of telemedicine programs are sensitive to these factors, they may be able to minimize certain problems at the outset as well as identify sources of problems that arise when the program becomes operational. The evaluation framework presented later in this report reflects this conclusion.

3

The Technical and Human
Context of Telemedicine

Telemedicine, like most other advanced information and communications technologies, depends on complex technical and human infrastructures that operate both within discrete institutions and across organizational and geographic boundaries. The individual components of these structures (e.g., tasks, roles, tools, procedures, and standards) are often quite complicated, and taken together their workings and effects may be exceedingly difficult to analyze and reconfigure.

In many respects, these complexities and difficulties are generic and are experienced by managers, technical personnel, workers, and consumers in business, education, government, and other arenas. Nonetheless, they must still be dealt with site by site and application by application as clinical uses of telemedicine are planned, implemented, evaluated, and redesigned. This chapter considers elements of the technical and human infrastructures that support clinical applications of telemedicine and that are often identified as the source of application failures or disappointments.

THE TECHNICAL INFRASTRUCTURE

Advances in the communications and information technologies that support telemedicine are so frequent, numerous, and complex that a thorough discussion of those that might be integral to a telemedicine evaluation would be both lengthy and partly out of date before it was even published. A recent "buyer's guide" issue of a telemedicine journal included nearly 50 pages of small-type tables listing product and service suppliers, products, and product specifications for video conferencing room systems, desktop video products, teleradiology products, and medical peripherals such as electronic stethoscopes, dental cameras, and video oto/ophthalmoscopes (Telemedicine Today, 1996). The service listing included telecommunications service providers, those offering telemedicine related services, and organizations providing other resources including telemedicine research and evaluation (see Table 3.1).

Overall, however, the health care sector has been described as relatively slow in adopting advanced communications and information systems. For example, a 1995 survey of 10 business sectors found health care respondents showing the lowest level of agreement that information networking was critical (35 percent compared to 48 percent for government and 71 percent for banking) and the lowest level of electronic information transfer (7 percent compared to 19 percent for government and 25 percent for business services) (NRC, 1996, p. 35). An earlier analysis of the growing use of telecommunications technologies likewise suggested that the health care sector has lagged somewhat behind other sectors of the economy in finding opportunities to substitute less expensive telecommunications for more costly capital, labor, and materials (Cronin et al., 1994).

Health care organizations are often only a small part of the market for various information and telecommunication technologies. Although technologies such as computed tomography and laser surgery were explicitly tailored to health care uses, other equipment and tools may not be designed with clinical uses and settings in mind—at least, initially. For example, expensive digital cameras produce the high resolution images needed for teledermatology, but some features, which were designed with newspaper and magazine photographers in mind, may be of marginal clinical value (Van Riper, 1996).

Furthermore, manufacturers may abandon technologies useful for some telemedicine applications because the total market is too limited to justify continued support of the product or because corporate realignments have shifted business priorities. For example, committee members heard military personnel express concern about the

TABLE 3.1 Types of Telemedicine Service Providers, Related Services, and Other Resources

Category	Type
Telecommunication service providers	Regional Bell operating companies Local exchange companies Independent operation companies Interexchange companies Competitive access providers Other
Telemedicine-related services	System design and integration Technical support/systems maintenance Value added network monitoring/management Telecommunications and telemedicine consulting Software systems design/provision Internet access services Other
Other telemedicine resources	Continuing medical education service providers Telemedicine research and evaluation organizations Medical information resources Telemedicine conferences/training Other

SOURCE: Adapted from *Telemedicine Today: Telemedicine Buyer's Guide and Directory*, Winter 1996 special issue.

possible discontinuation of Picasso, a basic, relatively inexpensive still-image phone system because it has not found a large enough market (Telemedicine Business Newsletter, 1995). From the radiology community, the committee heard some concern that picture archiving and communication systems (PACS) designed for digital image management on a large scale, are vulnerable to similar decisions by vendors concerned about returns on very expensive but slow-to-pay-off investments (Siegel, 1996; Ridely, 1996).

One other issue in the wider availability of telemedicine systems involves uncertainty about the regulation of medical software by the

Food and Drug Administration (Bashshur et al., 1994; OTA, 1995). Chapter 4 briefly reviews FDA policies on medical software and other medical devices used in telemedicine.

Table 3.2, which is taken from one of the last reports completed by the now defunct U.S. Office of Technology Assessment, lists key information technologies for health care (OTA, 1995). The list includes a highly varied mix of relatively discrete technologies (e.g., magnetic stripe cards) and more general concepts (e.g., clinical information systems). Although most have a potential, if not existing, place in one or another kind of telemedicine application, uses in banking, retail, entertainment, and other business areas may dominate technical, pricing, and related decisions for many of the discrete technologies such as hand-held computers. For telemedicine and for health care generally, computer-based patient records, clinical information systems, and clinical decision support systems—all of which involve management judgments as much as technical factors—are critical items on the list.

Variation in User Needs and Circumstances

Rural emergency departments, primary care clinics, public health facilities, correctional institutions, home care programs, and managed care plans may each need somewhat different technologies or combinations of technologies to fit their particular objectives and circumstances. As suggested by the examples in Chapter 2, real-time interactive audio and video connections may be essential in some situations, whereas telephone consultation may be quite satisfactory for others. In many cases, the relative effectiveness and costliness of different options remain to be systematically evaluated.

User needs or problems may also differ between the central service or consulting site and the site seeking the service or consultation. For example, a consulting radiologist or dermatologist may need a very sophisticated and expensive display unit that is capable of showing extremely fine gradations in images. For an attending physician, however, lower resolution may be sufficient to support discussions of an image with a consultant or with a patient. A central consulting site will need significant radiographic storage capacity whereas the remote site may need very little.

At both central and satellite practices, clinical and other staff must be trained (and trained anew as staff come and go and technologies change), space must be identified and adapted to handle new equipment, and backup arrangements must be made in case of system failures. Given the smaller patient base and limited resources of many satellite sites, these demands can impose significant burdens. For busy practitioners, the time for training can be hard to find. These problems suggest the paradox that the satellite locations most in need of the access benefits that telemedicine may provide may also find it particularly difficult to participate in telemedicine without major financial and other support.

Because different telemedicine applications may involve quite different combinations of technologies and because each telemedicine program reflects different organizational objectives and circumstances, the particular configurations of equipment and space will vary from place to place. Figure 3.1 depicts some of the components of a telemedicine consulting installation at National Naval Medical Center in Bethesda, Maryland. The equipment, which is employed in different kinds of consultations between the center and Naval Medical Clinic in Annapolis, Maryland, includes clinical and administrative work stations, communications and storage devices, and a variety of peripherals such as video cameras.

Variety and Complexity of Technologies

The variety and complexity of advanced technologies makes formidable demands on those responsible for planning, deploying, sustaining, and evaluating information and telecommunications systems and programs (see, e.g., IOM, 1991; OTA, 1995; NRC, 1996). These challenges arise from

1. the rapid pace of technological change affecting the hardware and software options;
2. the multiplicity of hardware and software options and pricing schemes;
3. the scarcity of standards to assure that different hardware and software options will work together well;
4. the requirements for specially adapted space, extensive user training and reinforcement, and sophisticated support staff;
5. the diversity of needs and circumstances among users within an organization; and
6. the need to develop a variety of communications links with

TABLE 3.2 Key Information Technologies for Health Care

Category	Technology
Human-computer interaction	Hand-held computers
	Handwriting/speech recognition
	Personal digital assistants
	Personal identifiers/fingerprint recognition
	Automated data collection
	Structured data entry
Storage, processing, compression	Computer-based patient records
	Magnetic stripe cards
	Smart cards
	Picture archiving and communications systems
	Medical imaging (radiology, pathology, other)
	Optical storage
	Image compression
	Digital signal processors
	Object-oriented software design
Connectivity	Clinical information systems
	Cabled, optical, wireless networks
	Internet and electronic mail
	World Wide Web
	Integrational Services Digital Network

"outside" organizations and individuals that differ in the capacities and configurations of their systems.

Evaluators, for example, may find the specific features of an application becoming outdated (or updated) or subject to significantly different pricing or marketing practices while they are still under investigation. Key aspects of the technical infrastructure of telemedicine that affect its feasibility, utility, and cost are briefly described immediately below. The discussion minimizes the use of more technical terminology, but the report's glossary provides definitions of some basic terms. The committee notes that the language of the National Information Infrastructure (NII) is subject to some dispute and flux. Terms that are commonplace in telemedicine discussions—such as "architecture," "multimedia," "interoperability,"

TABLE 3.2 Continued

Category	Technology
	Frame relay
	Asynchronous Transfer Mode
	Client-server computing
	Messaging and coding standards
	Proprietary and consensus standards
	Medical Information Bus Security
	Passwords
	Fault tolerant computers
	Redundant disk (RAID) systems
	Authenticators
	Encryption
	Firewalls
Data distillation	Decision support systems
	Pattern recognition
	Artificial neural networks
	Knowledge-based systems
	Relational databases
	Nomenclature/controlled vocabularies
	Knowledge discovery
	Natural language processing
	Encoders and groupers

SOURCE: Adapted from OTA, 1995.

and "network"—may be used and defined differently in different sectors of the NII (NRC, 1996).

Information Carrying Capacity

The capabilities of telemedicine are constrained by the information carrying capacity—the *bandwidth*—of the communications media on which they depend (e.g., copper telephone wires, coaxial cable). Bandwidth is expressed in hertz (Hz) units (the number of repetitions per second of a complete electromagnetic wave) or in bits per second (bps) units (a unit of information expressed in binary digits). Higher bandwidth tends to be more costly to install and maintain. Figure 3.2 illustrates the bandwidth requirements of dif-

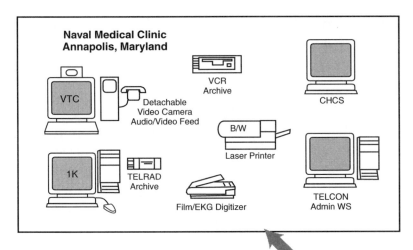

**Naval Medical Clinic
Annapolis, Maryland**

VTC

Detachable
Video Camera
Audio/Video Feed

VCR
Archive

CHCS

B/W
Laser Printer

1K

TELRAD
Archive

Film/EKG Digitizer

TELCON
Admin WS

T1 Transmission via landline

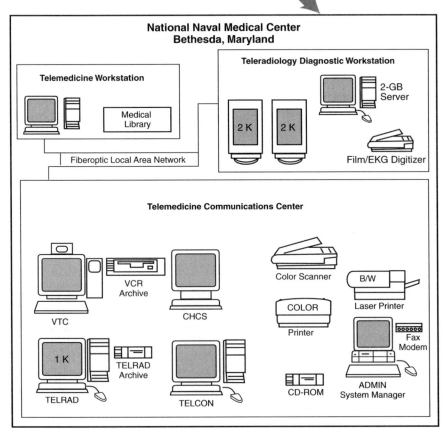

**National Naval Medical Center
Bethesda, Maryland**

Teleradiology Diagnostic Workstation

Telemedicine Workstation

Medical
Library

2-GB
Server

2 K   2 K

Fiberoptic Local Area Network

Film/EKG Digitizer

Telemedicine Communications Center

VCR
Archive

Color Scanner

B/W
Laser Printer

VTC

CHCS

COLOR
Printer

1 K

TELRAD
Archive

Fax
Modem

TELRAD

TELCON

CD-ROM

ADMIN
System Manager

ferent telemedicine applications and the capacity provided by different transmission media.

The costs and information carrying capacity of different telecommunications technologies are important because they affect the availability, quality, and affordability of information needed by clinicians to diagnose and manage health problems. Among the key dimensions of information relevant to physicians are

- sound fidelity;
- image resolution (spatial and contrast);
- range (completeness) of motion depicted; and
- transmission speed (or the amount of information that can be transmitted in a defined period).

In many respects, choosing among telemedicine technologies is an exercise in trade-offs involving the amount, quality, immediacy, and cost of different kinds of information. For example, satisfactory voice communication requires less bandwidth than satisfactory video communication, so decisionmakers must consider whether the cost of video technologies is worth the benefit in particular situations. Similarly, full-motion video useful for assessing gait or other physical signs is more demanding of bandwidth than common video conferencing technologies, which often show movement as somewhat jerky rather than smooth.

In nonurgent situations in which the patient remains in touch

---

FIGURE 3.1 Schematic representation of the telemedicine center at the National Naval Medical Center, Bethesda, Maryland and the satellite Naval Medical Clinic in Annapolis. ADMIN = administrative workstation; CHCS = Composite Health Care System (Department of Defense Hospital Information System); TEL CON = clinical video teleconferencing workstation; TELCON Admin WS = teleconferencing administrative workstation; TEL RAD = teleradiology workstation; TELRAD Archive = Picture Archiving and Communications Systems (PACS); T1 line = communications line capable of transmitting 1.544 Mbps of electronic information; VTC = video teleconferencing workstation; 2GB Server = two gigabyte server; 1K = standard resolution 1024 × 768 monitor; 2K = high resolution (for diagnostic imaging) 2048 × 1756 monitor. Sources: The NNMC-NMCL Annapolis Telemedicine Prototype Status Report prepared by Richard S. Bakalar for the Telemedicine Working Group, September 28, 1995; personal communication, R.S. Bakalar, July 2, 1996.

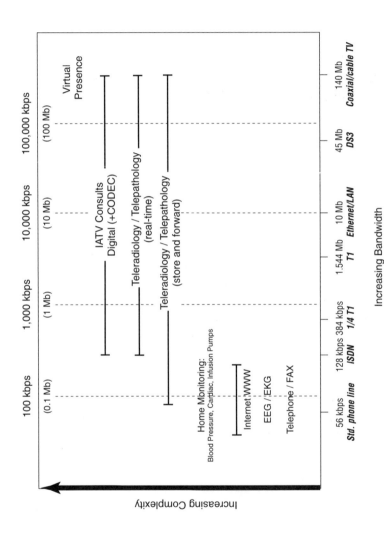

FIGURE 3.2 Relationship between the complexity of telemedicine applications and bandwidth (information carrying capacity) requirements (see glossary for explanation of terms and abbreviations). Source: Adapted from Allen and Perednia, 1996. Used with permission from *Telemedicine Today.*

with the primary care clinician, many consultations can be handled with good store-and-forward systems that allow still or video images to be sent to a remote data storage device from which they can be retrieved later and rerun. For example, a clinician or technician can transmit an image in the morning, but a distant consultant or technician can wait until that afternoon or evening to retrieve it. If such an arrangement suffices, then a system providing real-time images—and involving higher bandwidth and higher costs—need not be put in place. If, however, the patient is transient or otherwise unable to stay or return for the results of a consultation, then a real-time system may be appropriate. Real-time capacity is also appropriate for services dependent on extensive communication with the patient, most notably, telepsychiatry.

Once again, the demand for information carrying capacity depends on user needs and resources. Increases in capacity can be achieved by improving transmission media and by restructuring data. Both are briefly described below.

Information Transmission Media

Several different transmission media, with different capacities and costs, are available for telemedicine applications. Many telemedicine transmissions rely on telephone lines because they are so widely distributed and relatively inexpensive. Ordinary copper phone lines, however, have relatively low bandwidth (see Figure 3.2). Because they transmit large amounts of data relatively slowly, they are best suited for conventional telephone or for store-and-forward uses.

Enhanced copper phone lines can carry substantially more information per unit of time than ordinary lines for home phones, and fiber optic cable can provide even greater capacity. Use of these higher capacity technologies is expanding but is still constrained by the requirements for laying new lines, rewiring structures (e.g., hospitals, physician offices, homes), and installing other specialized equipment.

Coaxial cables, which already provide cable television to millions of households, also carry much more information than copper wires. Most cable systems are, however, structured for one-way rather than two-way communication and for home rather than business use. Although this is now a significant limitation on the use of existing cable networks to support certain kinds of home health services, changing technologies, costs, and regulations could alter the situation in a market that is highly competitive and volatile (Andrews, 1996).

Satellite and microwave systems offer additional options for transmitting very large amounts of data very quickly, but their high capital costs have made them unattractive for many telemedicine applications. They may, however, be the only transmission medium available for distant sites (e.g., ships, combat units) that cannot readily be reached by hard-wired systems. Also, if costs can be spread across other uses (e.g., for statewide educational networks as in the Oregon telepsychiatry program described in Chapter 2), then costs become more reasonable. At least one rural telemedicine program in Billings, Montana, rents time on its system to local businesses (Allen and Perednia, 1996; Dena Puskin, personal communication, May 10, 1996).

Because the prospective market for higher bandwidth is so lucrative, telephone, cable, computer, and other companies are competing on a number of fronts to achieve legal, technical, and other advantages. These fronts include the U.S. Congress, which recently passed major telecommunications legislation. Weekly if not daily articles in the financial press show that the federal telecommunications legislation passed in 1996 (see Chapter 4) is stimulating widespread reevaluation of strategies and alliances in the telecommunications industry. The implications for short-term and long-term advances in bandwidth options—and their stability—are likely to be significant.

Information Restructuring and Digital Technologies

Limitations on the carrying capacity of different transmission media can be overcome, in part, by restructuring or manipulating information before it is sent. In particular, the key to accurate and fast transmission of large amounts of information over long distances has been the development of techniques for converting continuous analog information or signals (e.g., sound waves, radiographs) into discrete digital signals coded in binary (e.g., on/off or 0/1) digits known as bits. The translation of data into digital form is also the foundation of other technological advances, most significantly, the computers that support the complex information processing requirements of modern communications technologies.

Some technologies further increase communications capacity by compressing data to reduce bandwidth requirements. This may or may not involve the loss of some information (and such loss may or may not be clinically important).

Digital data may also be packaged or manipulated in other ways. For example, packet switching technologies break digital data into small, standardized packets, several of which can be processed at once. This permits the fast transfer of large amounts of data.

The integrated service digital network (ISDN) is a protocol for standardized high-speed digital transmission of integrated audio, video, and data signals. It can be used with standard copper wires, but it requires installation of special digital input and output devices. The major benefit of ISDN is that it helps deal with the "last mile" problem of bringing high bandwidth into homes and offices without the high expense of rewiring them to connect with the rest of a telephone system that is mostly digital. In certain locales ISDN is available to residential as well as business customers, but marketing, pricing, service, fluctuating opinions about its value, and other problems have hindered its introduction (NRC, 1996).

The choice of specific techniques for coding, compressing, packaging, transmitting, and then decoding and displaying information may vary depending on several factors. These include the nature of the original signal (e.g., voice or video), the transmission distance, and the needs of users (e.g., for low versus high speed transmission or for moderately rather than highly accurate data). With the cost of some infrastructure options so high (e.g., laying cable to areas not currently served), financial considerations weigh heavily.

Making the Pieces Work Together

In any large health care organization, multiple information and communication systems initiatives may be under way simultaneously (IOM, 1991; Morrissey, 1996). The trend toward consolidation in health care delivery—including mergers of hospitals or health care systems and insurers, and purchase of physician practices and home care programs by hospitals—further complicates the information management picture as different information and telecommunications systems have to be understood and meshed. What two observers call the "hype associated with medical computing and telecommunications technologies" is, on the one hand, alluring to decisionmakers and, on the other hand, frustrating to those trying to distinguish real capacities from marketing hyperbole (Allen and Perednia, 1996, p. 9).

As described further in Chapter 7, the costs of a telemedicine application include up-front installation costs and continuing operating costs involving hardware, software, transmission, and support personnel. Misjudgments in the design and implementation of information and telecommunications systems are common and expensive, leaving organizations with perplexing decisions about whether (and for how long) the costs of replacing an unsatisfactory system exceed the costs of struggling to work with that system (NRC, 1996).

For managers at central telemedicine sites, some of the most frustrating aspects of telemedicine technologies involve how well the components operate together, work in different settings without extensive adaptation, and accommodate change (Bashshur et al., 1994; OTA, 1995). Phrased as questions, the issues are

- Is the hardware or software usable "off the shelf" or does it require custom design, fabrication, or programming?
- Does the hardware or software require considerable user sophistication or willingness to learn new procedures?
- Do the hardware or software components from different manufacturers (or even the same manufacturer) function together without difficulty?
- Do the hardware and software work together in modules that can be easily replaced when a component fails?
- When one component is replaced by a newer technology, will the new unit work with the remaining older components?

The problems implicit in these questions have led system users and major vendors to support modular components and open architecture, both of which make systems more flexible, adaptable, and easily maintained. Across the whole range of business and personal uses of information and telecommunications technologies, the persistent demand is also for more user-friendly systems. Among the critical ingredients for such systems are standards to link myriad different pieces of equipment and the software that makes them work.

Standards for Hardware and Software

The questions listed above highlight the issue of standards for designing hardware and software so that (a) different components of a telemedicine or other information and communication system work together (both within and across institutions) and (b) users can select compatible components from different vendors. Such standards cover a wide territory. For example, as characterized in one recent National Research Council (NRC) report,

> Standards describe low-level electrical and mechanical interfaces (e.g., the video plugs on the back of a television . . .). They define how external modules plug into a PC. They define the protocols, or agreements for interaction between computers connected to a common network. They define how functions are partitioned up among different parts of a system, as in the relationship between the television and the decoder now being defined by the FCC. They define the representation of information, in circumstances as diverse as the format of a television signal broadcast over the air and a Web page delivered over the Internet. [NRC, 1996, p. 151]

More than 400 private, mostly industry- or profession-specific organizations that develop standards are at work on information technology and telecommunications standards (NRC, 1996). In health care, a number of voluntary standard-setting groups and accrediting organizations for such groups have worked to develop standards in different areas including medicine, nursing, dentistry, and pharmacy. Figure 3.3 displays the array of messaging standards applicable to hospitals (OTA, 1995). Several organizations including the American Society for Testing and Materials (ASTM) and the American National Standards Institute, accredit standard-setting groups and also seek to coordinate the development of common approaches for messaging standards.

One major ongoing effort, Health Level Seven (HL7), which dates to 1987, develops standards for exchanging clinical, administrative, and financial information among hospitals, government agencies, laboratories, and other parties.[1] The HL7 standard covers the interchange of computer data about patient admissions, discharges,

---

[1]The term HL7 derives from the seven-part classification scheme for computer communications established by the International Standards Organization. The first level involves physical connections for equipment and the seventh involves messages.

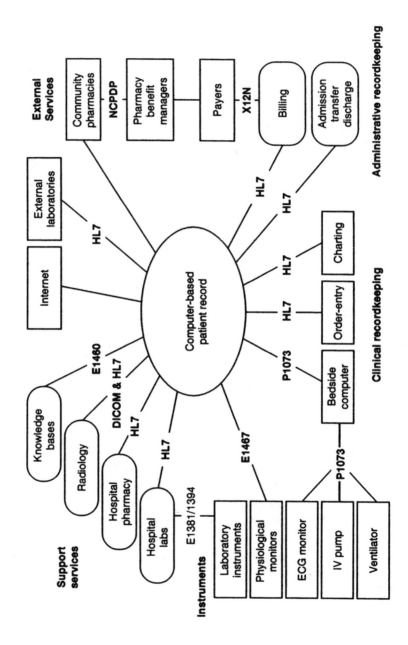

HL7
Standard for sharing clinical data written by Health Level Seven committee

E1381/1394
Standards for exchanging lab data among computers and instruments written by ASTM E31.14 subcommittee

P1073
Medical Interface Bus standard written by IEEE P1073 committee

E1460
Standard for sharing Modular Health Knowledge Bases written by ASTM E31.15 subcommittee

DICOM
Image exchange standard written by American College of Radiology and National Electrical Manufacturers Association

E1467
Standard for exchanging neurophysiological data written by ASTM E31.16 subcommittee

NCPDP
Pharmaceutical information exchange standard written by National Council of Prescription Drug Pharmacies

X12N
Insurance data exchange standard written by Insurance Subcommittee of Accredited Standards Committee X12

FIGURE 3.3 Messaging standards for electronic exchange of different kinds of hospital medical information. Source: OTA, 1995.

transfers, laboratory orders and reports, charges, and other activities. Most vendors of computer systems support this standard, which is also widely used internationally.

Radiology has been particularly active in standards development, dating back to the early 1980s. The American College of Radiology (ACR) and the National Electrical Manufacturers Association (NEMA) have cooperated to produce initial standards for exchanging digital radiological images and then to revise them in the face of changing technologies and user needs (ACR, 1994; OTA, 1995). The original standards emphasized connections between digital imaging equipment (e.g., a CT scanner) and display units and involved both hardware and software specifications. More recent work has focused on improving network communications capabilities and reducing hardware requirements. The major product as been the Digital Imaging and Communication in Medicine (DICOM) standard, which is now in its third version. A new working group has been considering whether and how to broaden the scope of DICOM by including other disciplines (e.g., cardiology, pathology) and other kinds of health information (ACR/NEMA, 1995).

Managing the Old and the New

A major issue for managers remains the rapid obsolescence—or at least succession—of hardware and software. Progress in information technologies often seems to comes in 18-to-36-month cycles that bring significant increases in processing speeds, storage capacity, or other technical dimensions. The advances that make systems faster, better, cheaper, more flexible, or convenient can be simultaneously satisfying and aggravating.

For example, as organizations move toward an integrated electronic patient record, they may not find it affordable or practical to replace all their older information systems for pharmacy, radiology, pathology, and other services. Thus, they often must develop innovative methods for connecting old, so-called "legacy" systems to new systems until it becomes possible to replace the old ones. In an increasingly competitive, cost-dominated environment, decisions about how much (and how) to invest in information technologies are both difficult and critical.

If the old systems have been abandoned by their manufacturers or software developers, finding replacement parts or qualified technicians, or even identifying software codes that need to be changed, may be difficult and expensive. The crises facing the nation's huge but obsolete air traffic control system dramatize this problem (Frey, 1996). Equally dramatic is the "millennium" or "year 2000" problem facing many banks and other major institutions that still rely in mundane but critical ways upon old, often undocumented software that cannot easily be changed to handle dates past the year 1999 (Duvall, 1996; IBM, 1996).

HUMAN FACTORS AND THE
ACCEPTANCE OF TELEMEDICINE[2]

The human infrastructure of telemedicine—like the technical infrastructure—is varied and complex. It generally will include an *intra*organizational and an *inter*organizational mix of clinicians (e.g., physicians and nurses), clinical support personnel (e.g., radiology technologists), physicists, engineering and computer specialists, administrative support personnel (e.g., appointment schedulers), and managers at consulting, satellite, or other sites. In addition, those directly involved in telemedicine will ordinarily be linked to other personnel involved in financial administration, information systems management, research, and a myriad of patient care activities.

Getting these human components—both individuals and organizations—to work well together and with complex and changing technologies is a never-ending challenge. By illuminating when and why these components are not performing as intended, evaluators can help program managers decide whether to continue, discontinue, or redesign operations and can also suggest to vendors and designers how their technologies might be better designed to accommodate human characteristics.

A major frustration with modern technologies is that while they promise to make life easier for people, they may simultaneously make it more difficult. Human factors engineer Donald Norman emphasized this in his book *The Design of Everyday Things:*

> We are surrounded by large numbers of manufactured items, most intended to make our lives easier and more pleasant. In the office we have

---

[2]This section is based on a background paper drafted by John C. Scott and Neal I. Neuberger.

computers, copying machines, telephone systems, voice mail, and fax machines. . . . All these wonderful devices are supposed to help us save time and produce faster, superior results. But wait a minute—if these new devices are so wonderful, why do we need special dedicated staff members to make them work—"power users" or "key operators"? Why do we need manuals or special instructions to use the typical business telephone? Why do so many features go unused? And why do these devices add to the stresses of life rather than reduce them? [Norman, 1990, p. vii]

The task of answering these questions (and seeing that they are asked) falls particularly within the domain of human factors engineering. This discipline seeks to design equipment, systems, and jobs by applying knowledge about how people interact with machines and how preferences and abilities affect these interactions (see, e.g., Salvendy, 1987; Rouse, 1991; Dumas and Redish, 1994; Gosbee, 1995). The issues raised and the strategies proposed by human factors engineers can inform designers and evaluators of telemedicine projects.

Growing Recognition of Human Factors

A recent overview of telemedicine technologies by two experienced telemedicine researchers argued that "most failures of telemedicine programs are associated with the human aspects of implementing telemedicine" (Allen and Perednia, 1996, p. 22). Similarly, in its site visits, meetings, and other activities, the committee heard repeatedly about the human factors that appear to underlie the rejection or limited acceptance of telecommunications and information technologies by otherwise interested clinicians and administrators.

Policymakers, too, have begun to appreciate that many of the programs which they have funded have used telemedicine far less than originally anticipated. For example, the federal Office of Rural Health Policy (ORHP), the Health Information and Applications Working Group of the Information Infrastructure Task Force Committee on Applications, the National Library of Medicine, and other agencies have sponsored a number of workshops and conferences on the opportunities and barriers facing telemedicine (see, for example, ORHP, 1993a; Bashshur et al., 1994, 1995; CPSC, 1995; Scott and Neuberger, 1996). Participants in these conferences have concluded, first, that much more research is needed to determine how patients and health professionals respond to telemedicine and, second, that the starting point for telemedicine should be the identification of needs and preferences of consumers and providers from a user- (e.g., patient, practitioner, community) rather than a technology-driven perspective. They also identified factors that may slow acceptance and adoption of telemedicine, including lack of documented benefit for clinicians; difficulty of incorporating telemedicine into existing practice; problems related to equipment; concerns about professional image; inadequate assessment of needs and preferences; lack of societal readiness; and health care restructuring (Scott and Neuberger, 1996).

To incorporate an examination of human factors, evaluators may in some cases be able to use program logs, debriefing interviews, or questionnaires to detect how these factors may have shaped the effects of telemedicine application. In other cases, they may infer the existence of certain problems based on their own experience, for example, their own frustrations with the technical limitations of hardware and software used in a particular application.

Although the research literature documenting the conditions for successful telemedicine programs is sparse, the conclusions above reflect a common view that telemedicine's successful transition from the demonstration phase into one of wide-spread use depends on better approaches to the human factors in telemedicine. The discussion below, which draws on the sources cited above, considers two broad categories of such factors: practical and socioeconomic. Users and potential users may also be discouraged by real or perceived policy barriers to telemedicine. Chapter 4 examines a number of such policies, including those that exclude payment for most consultations that are not provided on a face-to-face basis.

Practical Human Factors

Problems Related to Equipment

Telemedicine and information technologies are frequently "user unfriendly." Vendor sales, support, and other practices may also be frustrating and constraining. Among the problems reported to the committee were

- problems with the convenience, reliability, quality and integrity of equipment;
- lack of time to learn the correct use of complicated hardware or software that requires extensive training and continued reference to lengthy and highly technical user manuals;
- equipment purchase decisions based on grant and other financing requirements rather than appropriateness;
- lack of flexibility with proprietary systems;
- vendor restrictions on equipment leasing, which dictate large capital investment and maintenance costs for purchased equipment;
- constantly changing sales representatives and vendor product lines; and
- lack of market influence by small purchasers over vendors.

These problems are compounded when vendor marketing practices heighten clinicians' expectations about equipment performance and ease of use and then cannot deliver on their promises. Further, most product specifications and proposed technology solutions reflect the perspective of the technology vendor rather than the user of the product. More attention to applications-driven design, human factors engineering principles, and business process re-engineering might help to alleviate many of the problems identified here.

Difficulty of Incorporating Telemedicine into Existing Practice

When awkward, early stage telemedicine technologies and procedures are grafted piecemeal onto existing routines, the result can be important time management problems for clinicians and their patients. For example, interactive applications may require that primary care and consulting practitioners in different locations abide by the same schedule in order to use "real time" telemedicine systems. When managers in one telemedicine program charted the steps to schedule a telemedicine consult, they found it took at least 5 calls to do so and could take up to 25 calls (Armstrong, 1995). In contrast, much consultative medicine is practiced "asynchronously" with attending and consulting clinicians leaving messages for each other throughout the course of the day or over a period of days. Patients rather than data are often responsible for moving from place to place in the standard consultative medicine scenario. Computer-based scheduling programs can reduce though not eliminate scheduling

---

Box 3.1
Human Factors, Telemedicine, and the Telephone Analogy

In several respects, the current status of many telemedicine systems mirrors that of early telephone systems (Sanders, 1995). Earlier in this century, apartment buildings with 20 to 30 individual apartments typically had only one wall telephone on the ground floor for the entire apartment complex. When the phone rang, the hope was that a tenant in a nearby apartment would answer it and call to the phone the person being sought. This was inconvenient for all involved. Networking was inefficient and switching systems were slow; a person first had to reach an operator who in turn made a manual connection to another line. In addition, the sound quality was poor, maintenance was a problem, costs were high, and lines and equipment were scarce. Not surprisingly, telephone use was infrequent. The telephone only became indispensable when the communication infrastructure allowed for multiple, private lines in an apartment complex, so that each family had its own private line and could directly dial the party wanted.

---

problems, but the adoption of common or compatible systems across different organizations is not necessarily a simple step.

Another problem is the physical location of the telemedicine units, which are not always located where the services are being provided (e.g., a physician's office). In some cases, such an arrangement may seem reasonable, akin to having physicians go to the emergency room to see patients in urgent and emergency situations or having radiologists use special viewing rooms. More often, such an arrangement is artificial and inconvenient. Even if the equipment is only five or ten minutes away on another floor or in a nearby building, this can serve as a powerful deterrent to frequent use. Box 3.1 suggests parallels between the current status of tele-medicine systems and early telephone systems.

The widespread availability of practical and affordable desktop work stations should make it easier to employ telemedicine and a variety of other applications, such as patient record, clinical information, and decision support systems. Whether telemedicine or other applications are cost-effective for any specific user and situation still, however, would need to be assessed.

E-mail, voice mail, and fax machines—tools that are often overlooked as telemedicine technologies—may be better suited to some routine clinical communications, although improved store-and-forward technologies for data transmission should also permit for easier off-line consideration of information in response to medical requests.

In the future, clinicians could have available in one multimedia work station the capabilities, if needed, for visual (e.g., still images, full-motion video) and audio communication, graphics, medical literature searches, diagnostic peripherals, electronic mail, fax, and telephone. This technological base appears to be developing, pushed in considerable part by other service-oriented industries (e.g., entertainment, shopping, banking). The cost-effectiveness of telemedicine work stations, however, needs to be assessed, not assumed, for any given setting and set of uses.

A further issue involves the timely availability of relevant patient information. Clinicians involved in telemedicine consultations and other services often lack the whole picture, including patient history as well as current status and condition. Many health care institutions and most clinicians have not yet adopted computer-based patient records systems, but even those who have done so may find it difficult to integrate them with telemedicine applications. Barriers include the lack of common definitions and clinical vocabulary, inadequate standards for sharing and protecting the confidentiality of electronic data, and inconvenient documentation and data retrieval procedures. (In late 1996, the IOM plans to republish its 1991 report on the computer-based patient record with new commentaries describing developments since the original report was issued.)

Inadequate Assessment of Needs and Preferences

Given the discussion above, it is not surprising that a common criticism of advanced technologies is that developers and promoters too often fail to ask what practical needs or problems the technology might address. Even if such questions are asked, however, one dilemma in needs assessment is that "end users [in many instances] do not quite know what they want" and cannot readily imagine the uses of complex technologies with which they are often unfamiliar (NRC, 1996, p. 32). Thus, statements of provider or community needs may read like wish lists rather than realistic assessments and statements of priorities.

Needs assessments have several components. One involves the health status, problems, and other characteristics of the relevant population. A second relates to the characteristics, capacities, and objectives of individual practitioners and health care organizations. A third involves more broadly the characteristics and capacities of the health care system, including insurance coverage. User preferences may also be considered. For example, if color is preferred to black and white video, user aesthetic preferences may be relevant to decisionmakers considering video options. Even if a strategy may fail without such accommodation, financial considerations will undoubtedly affect the extent to which decisionmakers are willing to accommodate user preferences.

One pressing challenge is to develop methods and tools for assessing potential users' needs and for matching characteristics of particular telemedicine technologies to these needs. One study that attempted to determine clinicians' information needs employed a multidisciplinary evaluation team that (1) directly observed a randomized sample of clinicians for an eight-week period, (2) developed a process flowchart to identify process deficiencies and information requirements, (3) conducted semi-structured interviews, and (4) surveyed a larger group of clinicians to assess their experience with computers and their perceptions about the value of information system options (Tang et al., 1995). The results indicated not just a need for simple patient information but a need for information that was integrated, analyzed, and available when clinical decisions are actually being made.

Cultural and Socioeconomic Factors

Professional Culture and Image

Health care professionals take many of their cues from their colleagues. Thus, acceptance of a new technology by peers as well as opinion leaders may determine a clinician's receptivity to new practices. Most physicians have, however, developed referral patterns to specialists and subspecialists whom they know personally and see periodically on a face-to-face basis in professional or social settings. Telemedicine may disrupt this "culture" and perhaps damage local colleagues economically, as noted below.

In addition, appearances are important in the healing arts, and clinicians may be as concerned and self-conscious as anyone else about their appearance on camera. Because confidence is thought to be reassuring to patients and may, in and of itself, affect patient outcomes, clinicians may be concerned about the possibility that electronic media could weaken the patient's trust.

Nationally, because few programs have demonstrated sustained clinical and business benefits from telemedicine, role models are scarce. Evidence from other areas suggests that respected opinion leaders are important instruments of change because they serve as role models and trustworthy sources of information (or endorsement) for peer-oriented clinicians (Wolinksy, 1988; Soumerai and Avorn, 1990; IOM, 1992a). For those considering the introduction of a telemedicine program, the involvement of a range of specialists from a project's outset can help pave the way to acceptance by a broader community of colleagues.

Lack of Documented Benefit

The scarcity of rigorous evaluations of clinical telemedicine—the stimulus for this report—may also discourage clinicians and other decisionmakers. Little information is available to document how telemedicine can help health care organizations or clinicians improve health outcomes, promote better quality of care, manage costs, attract patients, reduce administrative hassles, or otherwise be of benefit. In addition, practitioners may be concerned that the early adoption of a new and relatively untested technology might be poorly regarded by the people they rely on for support and collaboration. A cautious approach to untested treatment modalities is generally expected of clinicians, and tolerance for "mistakes" in medicine is low. In time, recognized standards for telemedicine practice and direction from accrediting bodies may reduce this concern.

Absent an accessible body of knowledge to draw upon, clinicians and institutions must find their own paths anew. Journals, conferences, seminars, and Internet-based sources are beginning to fill the information vacuum, but the committee concluded from its sampling of these sources that more is sometimes promised than delivered by way of clear, accurate, and usable guidance. Moreover, in an era when health care institutions see each other as rivals not only within but also across communities, the climate for sharing information and experience is not always favorable.

Societal readiness is also an issue. Although some evidence suggests considerable patient acceptance of telemedicine in some settings (e.g., rural areas), it is not clear that patients are generally ready to accept that these new technologies will benefit them. The broader use of telemedicine may require, in addition to evidence relevant to clinicians and managers, efforts to inform and educate patients and consumers.

Lack of Payment for Telemedicine Services

Added to the uncertainties about the benefits of telemedicine is the important fact that most telemedicine consultations are not covered by Medicare or other third party payers (see Chapter 2 and Chapter 4 for additional discussion). Most of those interviewed by the committee believed this to be a major deterrent to telemedicine use, regardless of whether or not they were advocates of telemedicine or favored a change in payment policies.

Health Care Restructuring

Changes in the American health care system are altering the relationships between clinicians, patients, health care institutions, managed care plans, and public and private purchasers of health care. Strategic alliances, joint venture arrangements, and takeovers are changing historic relationships and centers of control over clinical practice. Practitioners and administrators are acutely concerned about protecting their patient base in the face of cost-driven reductions in the use of many services and changes in referral patterns. Advanced telecommunications technologies stand to alter further the relationships between health care organizations and professionals and between the practitioners and their patients. Will there be gatekeepers for telemedicine applications, and if so, who will play that role—clinicians, health plan managers, government officials, or perhaps the technicians who operate and maintain the equipment? For health care professionals accustomed to assigned roles and responsibilities, questions about who performs new and existing tasks in a networked environment may prompt considerable concern.

What may start as a simple way to improve access through telemedicine may end up as a permanent shift in the locus of patient care—locally, regionally, and even nationally. In the short term, this prospect may lead some to seek policy barriers (for example, licensure restrictions) or other limits on telemedicine practice. In the longer term, however, if telemedicine is viewed by managed care plans and integrated health systems as bringing cost and competitive advantages, they will use their leverage with government officials and employer purchasers of health benefits to implement telemedicine as they have done with other measures (e.g., discounted fees, utilization review) that are unpopular with clinicians.

CONCLUSION

Those responsible for creating, sustaining, and evaluating information and telecommunications systems and programs face a bewildering and constantly changing array of hardware and software options, many of which are not tailored to health care uses. Assessing the utility of advanced information and telecommunications technologies is difficult, particularly given the need to consider options in combination, not just individually. Although many groups are working to develop hardware and software standards, it remains frustrating and difficult to put together systems in which the components operate predictably and smoothly together, work in different settings without extensive adaptation, and accommodate replacement components.

Getting the components of the human infrastructure of telemedicine to function efficiently and predictably is also a major challenge. The limited adoption of telemedicine is due in part to a variety of what are commonly called "human factors," including a poor fit with the environment, needs, and preferences of clinicians, patients, and other decisionmakers (both individuals and organizations). Clinicians and other decisionmakers may be skeptical of telemedicine's clinical effectiveness as well as its practicality in everyday use. Thus, the scarcity of telemedicine evaluations and evidence of benefits is itself an element in the human factors equation. In addition, those advocating, adopting, or evaluating telemedicine must recognize the uncertainties and even fears that clinicians and organizations may have about how telemedicine will affect them in a period characterized by increased competition, structural realignments, and surpluses of some categories of health professionals.

This chapter has considered some elements of the technical and human infrastructures of telemedicine that evaluators may need to investigate if they are to provide assessments that help decisionmakers determine why a program succeeded or failed and whether and how it might be redesigned to work better. The next chapter considers some policy issues that evaluators may need to consider as they affect the adoption and implementation of telemedicine programs.

4

The Policy Context of Telemedicine

In their early days, most telemedicine programs had relatively low profiles politically. Clinical applications generally did not cross state borders, or if they did, they involved federal government agencies that were not bound by state licensure or liablity policies. The programs did not provoke much legal controversy at either the state or federal level, and decisionmakers, evaluators, and advocates did not appear immediately concerned with possible jurisdictional problems (Shinn, 1975).

Today, even though interstate telemedicine is not necessarily a high priority for many users or potential users, jurisdictional issues relating to licensure and medical liability are generating considerable debate and anxiety. Privacy and confidentiality have emerged as significant policy issues as computer-based patient information systems and databases have proliferated. Public and private policies regarding payment for telemedicine services are regarded by many advocates of telemedicine as a major obstacle. Whether and how such policy concerns are resolved can affect both the benefits and the costs of telemedicine and, thus, the sustainability of telemedicine programs.

At the same time that some governmental policies have posed problems for telemedicine, others have been devised specifically to encourage telemedicine. Such policies include demonstration project funding, technical assistance, research, and telecommunications infrastructure development that supports an array of applications, in particular, distance education.

Public policies, thus, present a mixed picture of incentives and disincentives for telemedicine that those contemplating telemedicine programs have good reason to examine carefully. Evaluators likewise may reasonably consider whether policy-related variables should be factored into evaluation plans. They may, for example, want to

- be alert for changes in a telemedicine program intended to achieve consistency with state or federal policies;
- enlarge the array of benefits, risks, and costs to be assessed;
- extend the search for possible determinants of telemedicine's acceptability, affordability, and even availability to clinicians, patients, and others; and
- investigate a broader range of practitioner or patient concerns about specific policy issues (e.g., privacy and confidentiality) to assess how well issues are understood and how important they are.

As additional context for the evaluation framework presented later in this report, this chapter examines several key policy issues. The first two sections briefly review federal and state initiatives to promote telemedicine either directly or as part of more general efforts to encourage communications and information technologies. The next three sections discuss professional licensure, malpractice, and the privacy and confidentiality of personal medical information. The final two sections consider telemedicine payment policies (a topic that covers both public and private actions) and the regulation of medical devices. Because it was not part of its charge, the committee did not make recommendations about the policy issues discussed here.

NATIONAL COMMUNICATIONS AND INFORMATION INFRASTRUCTURE POLICY

The most newsworthy recent federal action affecting telemedicine is the Telecommunications Bill of 1996, a broad and far-reaching reform of communications law that is expected to alter dramatically the telecommunications industry (Andrews, 1996). Among other changes, it allows long-distance telephone companies, cable companies, and other firms to compete with local phone companies, and local phone companies can, under some conditions, compete in the long-distance markets. Most rates for cable television will be deregulated within a period of three years.

Of greatest immediate relevance for telemedicine are provisions of the legislation directed specifically at assuring universal communications services at affordable rates for rural, high-cost, or low-income areas. One provision (Section 101 of the bill) states that "a telecommunications carrier shall . . . provide telecommunications services which are necessary for the provision of health care services in a State, including instruction relating to such services, to any public or nonprofit health care provider that serves persons who reside in rural areas" at rates comparable to those charged in urban areas. Telecommunications providers in rural areas are to be compensated through a fund designed to promote universal access to modern telecommunications services. This provision will be interpreted by regulations developed by the Federal Communications Commission. Other more general provisions of this major legislation may have quite significant implications for telemedicine, but their effects are difficult to predict very precisely at this early point.

Congressional interest in telemedicine is reflected in the Senate/House Ad Hoc Steering Committee on Telemedicine, which sponsors brown bag lunches and other events for members and staff interested in telemedicine. The group cosponsored a 1994 conference to develop a consensus agenda for telemedicine and health informatics (Bashshur et al., 1994).

During the 103rd Congress, at least 22 pieces of legislation specifically related to telemedicine were introduced (Telemedicine Monitor, 1995). Most explicitly or implicitly supported telemedicine in one way or another. In the first 15 months of the 104th Congress, telemedicine figured in at least 15 pieces of proposed legislation (Arent Fox, 1996). These proposals would, among other things, fund additional pilot projects, establish a commission on telemedicine, and include some telemedicine applications in health insurance reforms. Despite such positive signs, telemedicine was still targeted for a share of budget cuts as part of House and Senate proposals to eliminate the federal deficit.

More generally, as discussed in Chapter 1, telemedicine is just one element of a developing National Information Infrastructure (NII) that combines telecommunications and information technologies (Lindberg and Humphreys, 1995b). The White House has sponsored a major NII initiative to identify and resolve policy questions and speed the development and dissemination of information and telecommunications technologies not only in the government but also throughout the private sector in manufacturing, commerce, education, health care, and other areas.

An Information Infrastructure Task Force, led by the Department of Commerce, has the lead in coordinating activities related to the NII initiative. It created the Health Information Applications Working Group that, in conjunction with the Department of Health and Human Services, established the Joint Working Group on Telemedicine, chaired by the deputy director of the Office of Rural Health Policy (Puskin et al., 1995).[1] As discussed further in Chapter 5, one objective of that group has been to develop a broad evaluation framework for various federally funded demonstration projects and other telemedicine activities. The working group also has several additional areas of activity related to policy issues, safety standards, managed care, and development and maintenance of a telemedicine project inventory.

Another closely related federal enterprise is the High Performance Computing and Communications (HPCC) program (Lindberg and Humphreys, 1995a,b). This initiative emphasizes basic research and advanced technologies and networks. Some projects involve telemedicine and other health applications such as virtual reality tools for guiding or performing surgical procedures, computer-based patient records, and digital imaging software. These applications may raise a variety of regulatory issues, for example, FDA regulation of medical devices for safety and effectiveness.

In addition to these initiatives, several federal agencies have funded various kinds of demonstration projects intended to promote more specific agency agendas such as rural economic development. Appendix A provides information on several of these projects.

---

[1]The group includes representatives from various Cabinet departments, including Agriculture, Commerce, Defense, Health and Human Services, and Veterans Affairs, as well as from such other government units as Office of Management and Budget and the National Aeronautics and Space Administration.

STATE PROGRAMS AND INITIATIVES

Although some state policies or proposed policies have been viewed as barriers by those interested in making telemedicine applications less cumbersome, expensive, or risky, other state policies have directly supported telemedicine through legislation, demonstration funding, planning and coordination support, and other means (Lipson and Henderson, 1995; GAO, 1996). State initiatives in behalf of telemedicine have been concentrated in, but not limited to, the Midwest, Great Plains, and South. The objectives, scope, and depth of these initiatives are quite varied as are funding levels and sources. Some have focused primarily on medical education whereas others have emphasized service provision or support. The Western Governors Association (WGA) has expressed particular interest in initiatives to reduce some of the policy barriers to telemedicine described later in this chapter (WGA, 1995).

Evaluators need to be concerned about state initiatives, particularly as they may affect analyses of the cost, cost-effectiveness, convenience, or sustainability of telemedicine. For example, major infrastructure projects may provide a more enduring base for ongoing programs than do one-time grants.

As recently as 1992, only five states had explicit telemedicine planning or development efforts. According to a study undertaken by the Intergovernmental Health Policy Program (IHPP), the number was at least three times that in 1995, and additional states were considering action (Lipson and Henderson, 1995). The IHPP study, which covered 28 states, grouped states into five categories: (1) those with relatively well-developed state programs; (2) those with less well-developed programs; (3) those on the verge of program development; (4) those with some activities but no program; and (5) those with little or no state presence. Table 4.1 presents these categories with illustrative examples of state activities.

Some states surveyed by the IHHP have active telecommunications programs to support rural schools and libraries, but they have not made medical linkages a state policy priority. For example, a recent General Accounting Office (GAO) report profiled three states, two of which, Iowa and North Carolina, have encouraged medical care as well as educational links whereas the third, Nebraska, has emphasized educational links by the University of Nebraska Medical

TABLE 4.1 Categorization of 28 State Telemedicine Programs in 1995 with Examples

Program Category	States
Relatively well-developed	Georgia, Kansas, Louisiana, South Dakota, Texas

Example: "Telemedicine has had a very evolutionary development in Texas. . . . Texas has funded several . . . telemedicine and distant learning projects while support for telemedicine has been building in the state's academic health centers and the state prison system. . . . [Public utilities legislation] promises to create a statewide telemedicine and distance learning system with the largest funding [from private telecommunications companies] ever available in a state. . . . As of 1995, the state is taking a very aggressive role in telemedicine." (p. 1-13)

Less well-developed	Iowa, North Carolina, Oklahoma, Oregon, Pennsylvania

Example: "Apart from first establishing a network for distance learning that has been used for health applications, [Oregon's] role has been largely limited to funding for one specific program. However, Oregon, like the other states, has now taken action to establish a central planning role for all telecommunications. This action was necessary because of limitations in the current telecommunications infrastructure." (pp. 1-14 and 1-15)

Near development	Arkansas, New Mexico, Utah

Example: "Utah launched into program development with no state planning. However, Utah has a range of technology and telecommunications activities that may lead to a more coordinated role for the state." (p. 1-15)

Activities but no program	California, Colorado, Kentucky, Virginia, Washington, West Virginia, Wyoming

Example: "Virginia's authorization of a study on telemedicine may be a prelude to further state involvement." (p. 1-15)

Little or no activity	Arizona, Florida, Idaho, Maine, Minnesota, Montana, Nebraska, Ohio

NOTE: A number of the 22 states not categorized do have some policies or activities related to telemedicine.

SOURCE: Lipson and Henderson, 1995.

Center, which was the site of some of the earliest medical education experiments with telemedicine, as described in Chapter 2 (ORHP, 1993b, and GAO, 1996).

In addition, some states not surveyed for the IHHP study do have some level of state support for telemedicine. For example, the state of Maryland's trauma system includes telemedicine applications, which were discussed with the committee during a site visit. More states can be expected to develop policies on telemedicine in the future.

PROFESSIONAL LICENSURE AND DISTANCE MEDICINE

Telemedicine challenges the traditional view of professional practice as involving a face-to-face encounter between clinician and patient. This encounter made "the place where medicine was practiced, and who was practicing, . . . obvious" (Gilbert, 1995b, p. 28). Telemedicine breaks that physical link and thus complicates decisions about where a telemedicine practitioner should be licensed if the practitioner and patient are located in different states.[2]

Many telemedicine programs are not affected by these complications because they operate entirely within a single state. In addition, telemedicine programs operated by the federal government are not restricted by state licensure laws. For example, clinicians and managers working in the military, the Department of Veterans Affairs, the U.S. Public Health Service, and the federal prison system can proceed with cross-state tests and applications of telemedicine without concern about state challenges or penalties.

Current Policies

In the United States, the responsibility for licensing and otherwise regulating health professionals lies with state governments. States originally adopted licensure laws and objective criteria for entry into designated health professions to protect people from charlatans and untrained individuals holding themselves out as qualified

---

[2]This discussion draws on Gilbert, 1995a,b,c; Granade, 1995a,b,c; McIlrath, 1995a; Young and Waters, 1995. In addition, Francoise Gilbert (letter, March 25, 1996) and Leo Whalen (letter, March 24, 1996) reviewed the text and made a number of helpful suggestions.

medical personnel. All states require physicians, nurses, dentists, and certain other health care personnel to be licensed by the state to practice their profession. The penalties for practicing medicine without a license are significant and may include criminal as well as civil penalties.

State laws, which were adopted long before the advent of modern telemedicine, also require any out-of-state physician who diagnoses or treats a patient in the state to be licensed in that state. Most states, however, provide an exception that allows physicians licensed in that state to consult with the licensed physicians from other states (and sometimes other countries). This exception is intended to allow patients to have access to the talents and expertise of physicians from other states without having to travel to those states.

State consultation exceptions are not uniform. Some exceptions are broadly stated, but others limit the exception to one-time or occasional consultations or include other restrictions. Generally, consultation provisions do not appear to offer protection for an out-of-state clinician unless a consultation is requested by or otherwise involves an in-state clinician. A few states, including Louisiana and Pennsylvania, do not have an explicit consultation exception.

Recently, some states have amended or are considering amending their physician licensing statutes (or changing the interpretation of existing statutes) to prohibit out-of-state physicians from practicing without a license in that state (Gilbert, 1995b; Young and Waters, 1995; Richardson, 1996).[3] Indiana, Texas, South Dakota, and Nevada have enacted statutes that require out-of-state telemedicine providers to be licensed in those states. The Texas statute states that "a person who is physically located in another jurisdiction but who, through the use of any medium, including an electronic medium, performs an act that is part of a patient care service initiated in this

---

[3]Such restrictions have also been aimed at utilization management programs that require that proposed hospitalizations or medical procedures be reviewed or certified in advance as "medically necessary" to qualify for insurance coverage. Many of these programs are operated by national or regional firms that concentrate in one or a few locations the physicians, nurses, clerks, or other personnel who review or certify services for coverage. The contention is that these activities, especially when coverage is not certified, constitute the practice of medicine, and, therefore, they must be undertaken by physicians licensed to practice within the state in which the patient resides (Field and Gray, 1989; Gosfield, 1991).

state . . . and that would affect the diagnosis or treatment of the patient, is engaged in the practice of medicine in this state for the purposes of this Act" (Texas HB 2669, amending the Texas Medical Practice Act, Article 4495b of the Texas Civil Statutes). The amended statute does not contain a narrow exception for "episodic" consultations with physicians in the same medical specialty.

Other states, such as Florida, have narrowed statutory consultation exceptions by administrative regulation or by interpretation. In a widely cited action in May 1994, the Kansas Board of Healing Arts adopted a regulation requiring that—except as authorized by statute—any person "regardless of location" must be licensed in Kansas if he or she "treats, prescribes, practices, or diagnoses a condition, illness, ailment, etc., of an individual who is located in Kansas" (Kansas Regulation 100-26-1). The Kansas legislature, however, has not amended the statutory consultation exception (Kansas Statute 65-2802), which exempts from licensing out-of-state physicians engaged in the healing arts in consultation with a licensed Kansas physician. Thus, the effect of the Kansas regulation is not entirely clear.

Restrictive state positions have been challenged by those who argue that a telemedicine service involving an out-of-state clinician does not involve the practice of medicine in the state where the patient is located. In this view, the situation is simply equivalent to a medical visit for which the patient travels physically rather than electronically to another state. To date, this perspective has not prevailed.

If a reliance on state consultation provisions does not appear possible or prudent and if a telemedicine practitioner believes it necessary or sensible to seek licensure in other states, the requirements for doing so will vary from state to state. Some states provide for licensure by endorsement, which means they will grant a license to a clinician already licensed by another state with equivalent or stricter requirements. Licensure by endorsement may not, however, be easy. For example, South Carolina requires "a fee; two photos; an application completed in part by the physician's medical school, the state or national board which issued the original certificate by written exam, and if possible a medical society; the signatures of three South Carolina licensed physicians if at all possible; and a personal appearance by the applicant before the medical board" (Granade, 1995a, p. 6).

Issues

Why do licensure requirements create problems for clinicians and organizations involved in telemedicine practice across state lines? First, obtaining a professional license involves some expense, including initial and renewal licensing fees. Some states require a face-to-face interview, which entails expenses for travel.

Second, obtaining and maintaining multiple licenses can involve considerable time, research, and paperwork, which may, in turn, involve additional expenses (Collins and Charboneau, 1993). Because requirements for licensure vary from state to state, new analyses have to be undertaken and new forms completed for each state in which a clinician expects to provide telemedicine services. Moreover, requirements for maintaining a license also vary with respect to the time intervals for relicensure, provisions for continuing medical education, and other matters.

Third, licensure typically brings with it a number of obligations with which clinicians must be familiar. Although broadly similar, state laws may vary on specific points, such as confidentiality requirements (Eid, 1995). For example, Colorado and Minnesota "require doctors to disclose to the state the names of HIV-positive patients' sexual partners, [while] New York and California say those names can't be disclosed" (Richardson, 1996, p. A8). California gives individuals the right to review their medical records, but Maryland does not (Eid, 1995). What would be the situation of a Maryland patient with a California telemedicine consultant?[4]

Many of the current practical burdens of multiple licensure could be eased for individual practitioners if health care institutions assisted with expenses and provided administrative support as costs of doing business. Moreover, the development of national practitioner databases should make access to information about physicians much easier, although concerns about the accuracy and importance of included data have made such databases controversial. Nonetheless, the ultimate responsibility for adhering to licensure requirements resides with the clinician.

---

[4]Further complicating the legal picture for telemedicine practitioners and programs is the still unresolved question of where a telemedicine patient's records should be kept (e.g., at the distant consultant's office or the local attending's office) and in what form (Gilbert, 1996).

(R&D) resources; integrated medical records and better access to follow-up data on patients; and a command structure that can promote cooperation across diverse sites. As a major purchaser of information and communications technologies, the military also has the leverage to stimulate the development of better vendor data on the effectiveness and costs of relevant hardware and software.

The initial DOD work has focused on evaluation strategies and tools and early "proof of concept" and description evaluations. For example, during U.S. operations in Somalia in 1993, the Army tested several technical, clinical, and administrative components of a new telemedicine support system for troops deployed in military or peacekeeping missions. A model is being developed to define medical specialty requirements for deployed troops, but it should also be applicable during peacetime.

Department of Veterans Affairs

Like the military, the health care system operated by the Department of Veterans Affairs (VA) has characteristics that are attractive to those evaluating telemedicine. In addition, the VA has, over several years, developed a fairly comprehensive and flexible patient information system that can integrate text, test results, and images in a computer-based patient record (Dayhoff, 1996).

Taking advantage of the system's health services research capacity and its link with academic medical centers, clinicians at a number of medical centers are already engaged in or planning evaluations of various clinical applications of telemedicine. For example, this chapter cites activities involving the VA Medical Centers in Baltimore and Palo Alto.

The committee learned that a task force had proposed a coordinated telemedicine evaluation strategy for the Department of Veterans Affairs but that no decision had been made to adopt and implement it. The department has, however, moved to inventory the system's telemedicine activities. Results indicate that most VA Medical Centers (VAMCs) either have some kind of operational telemedicine program or are planning one (VA, 1996). Beyond ordinary telephone-based consultation and triage, the most common clinical application appears to be teleradiology. Interest in telemedicine applications is likely to grow as a result of recent policies to shift more care from inpatient to outpatient settings and to encourage more regional coordination among medical centers (McAllister, 1996).

Health Care Financing Administration

As part of a continuing initiative to evaluate telemedicine and inform Medicare coverage policies, the Health Care Financing Administration (HCFA) has supported a number of projects intended to provide general guidance for telemedicine evaluations as well as data on the effects of particular applications of telemedicine. Two of these projects are described immediately below. A third (involving the University of Michigan and the Medical College of Georgia) is described later.

Center for Health Policy Research

In 1993 and 1994 with support from HCFA, Grigsby and his colleagues at the Center for Health Policy Research (CHPR, which is affiliated with the Center for Health Services Research and the University of Colorado Health Sciences Center) presented a series of four reports on telemedicine (Grigsby et al., 1993, 1994a,b,c). (Their specific research projects are described later in this chapter.) HCFA asked the CHPR to develop an evaluation framework and a general strategy for assessing the effects and effectiveness of telemedicine. The key components of the framework included

- a conceptual framework with three dimensions (technological adequacy, medical effectiveness, and appropriateness);
- a taxonomy and classification of telemedicine applications; and
- recommendations for telemedicine research on medical effectiveness, cost, access, utilization, acceptance, payment, and related issues.

The researchers noted that although telemedicine is more than simply hardware and software, "a crucial aspect of the conceptual framework . . . is the delineation of a method for establishing minimally acceptable system parameters and standards for hardware and software" (Grigsby et al., 1993, p. 3.2). Such evaluations can provide important information for those responsible for developing national and international standards, as described in Chapter 3. Technological adequacy was not directly defined but informally described as whether a technology is "good enough for now" for the intended purposes and circumstances. The researchers argued that evaluators need better strategies for assessing the adequacy of the

- input data—including its quality (e.g., image resolution, sound quality), the speed of the equipment for encoding and delivering it to the main transmission medium, and the quality of any data compression and other pretransmission modification of the data;
- transmission of data—based on the bandwidth (information carrying capacity) of the communications medium, its cost, and practicality; and
- display of data received—including the quality of the images, sound, or other information, and the options for enhancing or otherwise manipulating the information (e.g., increasing or decreasing contrast).

The CHPR discussion of medical effectiveness is consistent with the definition offered in Chapter 1 (results under normal conditions of use) and emphasizes the need for comparison with conventional services. The discussion focuses on practical strategies such as (a) narrowing the range of conditions and indicators of effectiveness to be studied; (b) establishing minimal levels of diagnostic accuracy for particular applications and conditions; and (c) assessing the appropriateness (a combination of effectiveness, cost-effectiveness, and acceptability to patients and physicians) of using a technology in specific health care environments (e.g., rural areas) and for specific clinical problems and types of patients (e.g., gynecological examinations).

The proposed taxonomy sorted telemedicine applications according to the level of evidence or consensus about their effectiveness, a key criterion for coverage. Applications or aspects of evaluations can be described as (a) effective; (b) probably effective; (c) not demonstrated as safe and effective; or (d) new and untested.

For purposes of HCFA coverage policy (as governed by statutes and regulations), even the first category—applications that are judged effective—may raise additional questions about implementation and economic impacts that warrant pilot tests designed to guide explicit coverage decisions and monitoring strategies. Examples of such questions include how to structure supervision, consultations, and payments for nonphysician primary care providers in remote sites. The "probably effective" category of applications generally has not been the subject of full-fledged evaluations that describe basic characteristics of the applicants' implementation and impact. Telepsychiatry falls into this category. The third category (not demonstrated as safe and effective) includes applications for which procedures or standards for safe and effective use have not been established or sufficiently refined to warrant routine use. For example, in radiology, some consider the safety and effectiveness of digital mammography inadequately documented, although the technology is being employed on a limited basis already. The final category of new and untested technologies includes those that are clearly experimental such as remote surgery.

Grigsby more recently suggested that three coverage-relevant categories would be sufficient: (1) effective; (2) probably effective but with unknown effect on the health care system (e.g., increased costs); and (3) not demonstrated as effective (and with serious ramifications if ineffective) (personal communication, March 7, 1996). In addition, in a recent article, Grigsby and colleagues proposed three key questions for evaluation (Grigsby et al., 1995, pp. 126–127): (1) Are specific telemedicine applications medically effective means of delivering health care? (2) What are the costs involved in specific telemedicine applications, and are these applications cost-effective means of providing health care? (3) What processes of telemedicine are associated with optimal health outcomes? The group also proposed two key policy questions: (4) Can appropriate use be defined? and (5) How should payment for telemedicine services be handled?

Telemedicine Research Center

One of the problems in evaluating telemedicine applications is the small number of cases generated by most demonstration or pilot projects (Crump and Pfeil, 1995; Perednia, 1995). The Telemedicine Research Center, an independent, nonprofit organization located in Portland, Oregon, has created a Clinical Telemedicine Cooperative Group (CTCG) to promote the pooling of information from multiple telemedicine evaluations (Perednia, 1996). Taken as a whole, the center's work includes both elements of an evaluation framework (e.g., generally applicable concepts and protocols) and actual evaluations (e.g., compilation and analysis of data).

Working from a model provided by cooperative oncology research networks and with funding from HCFA, the CTCG involves subscribers (e.g., research projects) who are permitted to use the research tools (e.g., questionnaires) developed by the group in exchange for a small subscription fee and an agreement to contribute their data for aggregation and analysis (Perednia, 1995). The subscribers' research projects should have some common components (e.g., certain questions asked of patients), although they might differ in other respects.

Such efforts need to assess when data (e.g., patient satisfaction, utilization rates) can be meaningfully aggregated for disparate applications or when the data are meaningful only if like uses are pooled. The latter category includes information on accuracy rates for specific diagnoses or outcomes for specific clinical applications. For a multisite cooperative evaluation effort, these different situations affect the choice of questions asked and the way responses are analyzed. Obviously, questions about characteristics of a skin lesion make no sense for telepsychiatry sites. On the other hand, questions about clinician acceptance of a technology might be analyzed in pooled form (i.e., for disparate programs) as well as for distinct applications (e.g., for teledermatology visits only or for just the store-and-forward teledermatology data). Researchers also should be sensitive to limits on pooling data created by other differences in research design and methods. These limits have been discussed in the context of growing use of formal meta-analyses (see, e.g., Eysenck, 1994; Greenland, 1994; Bailar, 1995).

The Telemedicine Research Center also sponsors an on-line computer information service, collaborates with other researchers, and develops tools to support telemedicine evaluations.[3] One of these tools is the Evaluation Question Hierarchy and associated software, which are designed to generate specific questions tailored to particular research problems, to streamline the process of questionnaire

---

[3]The Telemedicine Information Exchange (TIE) can be found on the Internet at http://tie.telemed.org/. It provides links to many other telemedicine information sites sponsored by governmental, university-based, commercial, and other organizations. In early 1996, it had about 300 Internet sites linked to it.

construction so that researchers do not have to start anew on each project, and to encourage efforts to pool data from multiple projects. The software links four kinds of factual questions to several policy questions (e.g., was a program cost-effective?). They attempt to identify

- what happened in association with the intervention or control situation;
- what the financial impact was;
- what the clinical impact was; and
- how participants reacted.

EXAMPLES OF INDIVIDUAL RESEARCH STRATEGIES

This chapter began by noting the dearth of rigorous evaluations of clinical telemedicine. Although this study was intended to develop an evaluation framework rather than to draw conclusions about the effectiveness of telemedicine, the committee did search for research overviews and published reports that might provide models or lessons for its work. Most of the reports it reviewed focused on technical quality or feasibility (what was termed above "test of concept" studies) with few addressing effects on health outcomes, process of care, access, or costs.

The literature reviews consulted by the committee include extensive reviews conducted by the Center for Health Policy Research under its contract with the Health Care Financing Administration (Grigsby et al., 1993, 1994a,b,c; Grigsby et al., 1995) to determine whether the literature "supported the use of telemedicine as a safe, medically effective set of procedures" (Grigsby et al., 1995, p. 116). The investigators found relatively few peer-reviewed studies, only a limited amount of work in progress, and a highly varied mix of research approaches and targets with no replications or cross-validating studies (Grigsby et al., 1995, p. 117). Another review of the literature by Sanders and Bashshur yielded similar conclusions: "Much of the appeal [of telemedicine] remains intuitive and based on fragmentary rather than systematic empirical research" (Sanders and Bashshur, 1994, p. 7).

The committee's review of the literature was designed primarily to identify different research strategies and useful research tools. Unfortunately, this review experienced the same difficulties found by the substantive literature reviews, that is, a modest research base, limited documentation of methods, and research designs changing during implementation. Nonetheless, the committee reviewed a number of planned or completed projects and selected several as illustrative of the more rigorous approaches taken by some investigators. These projects are briefly described below with an emphasis on their purposes, designs, and difficulties.

Studies to Compare Digital versus Conventional Images

Perhaps the largest quantity of systematic comparative telemedicine research has dealt with medical images viewed on electronic workstations compared to conventionally viewed images (e.g., radiology films, glass pathology slides) or direct patient examination, for example, of skin lesions. Researchers in radiology, in particular, have accumulated considerable experience in evaluating the quality of digital imaging and image transmission compared to the "gold standard" of conventional film images (Grigsby, 1995a).

Early studies in the 1970s and 1980s generally found that images produced via teleradiology were not of acceptable quality compared to film images (Gitlin, 1986; Grigsby et al., 1993). More recent research employing improved equipment is producing good results for a variety of uses, and researchers are continuing to explore the strengths and limitations of teleradiology for specific clinical problems, settings, and purposes (see, e.g., Decorato et al., 1995; Mun et al., 1995; Roponen et al., 1995; Wilson and Hodge, 1995).

Work at Johns Hopkins University illustrates the shift in research results. In an initial effort to assess the acceptability of digital images for primary interpretation by emergency department physicians, researchers selected images from their radiology library based on their clinical importance and difficulty and also selected a comparison group of less challenging images (Scott et al., 1995). Based on comparisons involving four different groups of readers (staff radiologists, emergency physicians, radiology residents, and emergency medicine residents) using the relatively low resolution monitors then available, they concluded that the teleradiology images were not satisfactory for primary interpretation. Later work at the same institution using the same general strategy described above but employing more advanced equipment for digitally producing, transmitting, and displaying images (in particular, higher resolution monitors) has

shown agreement for primary diagnosis between film-based interpretations and those done using electronic work stations (Gitlin,
1996).

The contrast in results for the earlier and later studies of teleradiology underscores the difficulties of conducting research—and
making technical, clinical, and financial decisions about equipment
and software purchases—when technologies are changing and improving rapidly. The committee understands that the major debates
about the quality of digital images in radiology now involve mammography, subtle skeletal problems, and some pulmonary applications (Mun et al., 1995; Wilson and Hodge, 1995). According to
one expert, "what now needs major assessment is the effect of
teleradiology on patient management and outcome," including the
timeliness of care and cost-effectiveness (Franken, 1996).

Some work is under way to assess the impact of digital radiology
systems on productivity. At the Baltimore Veterans Affairs Medical
Center, investigators collected baseline data for three months before
implementation of their institution-wide digital imaging system and
then collected data again after the system had been in place for a
year (Siegel, 1996). The results indicated that although it took a
radiologist about 40 percent more time to use a computer work
station rather than a conventional viewing system set up by technicians, overall productivity increased by about 25 percent. The investigators attributed this increase to several factors, including better
workload sharing, home access to images, fewer interruptions,
quicker and more organized access to previous images and reports,
and elimination of time spent waiting for film to be developed. The
time between taking an image and its interpretation also dropped.
Survey information suggested that other clinicians were consulting
less with radiologists because they had "bedside access" to images,
and this led to steps to encourage such consultations.

Dermatologists and pathologists have also been active in imaging research (see, e.g., Krupinski et al., 1993; Perednia and Brown,
1995; Barnard and Middleton, 1995; Menn and Kvedar, 1995;
Seykora, 1995). This work has involved not only the comparison of
digital and conventional images but also the comparison of video
and still images and the comparison of images with direct physical
examination.

Dermatologists use color and texture information in diagnosis,
and the requirements for diagnostic quality color images are still

being explored.[4] The committee's site visits turned up two image evaluation studies in dermatology. A project at the Oregon Health Sciences University (with assistance from the Telemedicine Research Center and funding from the National Library of Medicine) is intended (a) to verify that electronic images can be used to make accurate diagnoses and (b) to determine the minimum technical specifications required for the capture of diagnostically relevant information (Perednia and Brown, 1995). Clinical photographs with proven diagnoses will serve as the "gold standard" against digital images acquired, transmitted, or stored under varying conditions (e.g., different video formats, different color resolution). In another project, Stanford researchers will compare image quality for three groups of patients: one involving real-time video consults; a second using store-and-forward video technology using technicians to acquire the images; and the third relying on face-to-face examinations (Barnard, 1995).

Evaluations of Automated, Telephone-Based Services

As noted in Chapter 2, nonvideo applications of telemedicine are common in the form of telephone calls initiated by patients or clinicians. A variety of telephone-based computer-assisted services have also been developed over more than two decades (see, e.g., Greenlick et al., 1973; Muller et al., 1977; Alemi and Stephens, in press). These include automated systems that call to remind people of scheduled appointments, programs that provide recorded health information, and others that monitor patient status and record voice answers or touch-tone telephone responses.

Alemi and colleagues at Cleveland State University have reported on a number of attempts to use quasi-experimental research designs to evaluate the effectiveness of these kinds of services. One study

---

[4]The problem of color fidelity is familiar to amateur photographers and television viewers. The committee heard anecdotes about physicians worried about the pale color of patients seen in video consultations who discovered the problem was with their color monitor. In a study reported in 1977 that compared on-site physician diagnoses with remote physician diagnoses using telephone, still-frame black-and-white television, black-and-white television, and color television, few differences were found among the telemedicine options (Dunn et al., 1977). For dermatology diagnoses, however, telephone did worse (as expected) but so did color television because of color inaccuracies.

examined a telephone-based health risk assessment program designed to inform students about their risk levels for blood pressure, seat belt use, and other factors. Evaluators first randomly selected and interviewed control subjects prior to the introduction of the program and then randomly selected experimental subjects to participate in the program (Alemi and Higley, 1995). The sequence was designed to avoid contamination of the control subjects because once the experimental program was available it could be shared with those who were not part of the formal test group. Those in the test group who used the program (71%), when interviewed later, reported higher satisfaction with the experimental system than the control group reported for their current sources of health information. The experimental group, however, reported that the risk information was redundant in that they were already aware of their status on most risk factors.

Another study of an automated monitoring system did not employ randomization but rather used a single-group time-series design that provided for weekly computerized telephone interviews over a nearly five-month period and also for mail surveys during the 4th, 10th, 14th, and 18th weeks (Alemi et al., 1994). Response rates for the telephone interviews were higher than for the mailed surveys (1994).

In a third study, investigators randomly assigned pregnant patients with a history of drug use to participate in experimental and control groups (Alemi and Stephens, in press). Both groups received certain services including case management and obstetrical care. The experimental group also received a variety of telephone-based computer-assisted services including information and support services using automated reminder and other calls, conference calls, and voice mail arrangements. A forthcoming issue of the journal *Medical Care* is being devoted to reports on this third set of studies.

Describing Deployment Telemedicine

As discussed earlier in this chapter, the Department of Defense has been working to develop a coherent evaluation strategy for telemedicine. It has already accumulated considerable practical experience in telemedicine consultations involving a number of its major medical centers. The experience with deployed troops was recently described in an article by Walters (1996). She retrospectively analyzed all 171 telemedicine consultations received from deployments in Somalia, Macedonia, Croatia, and Haiti between February 1993 and March 1995.

In this study, a third of the records were excluded for lack of key data (e.g., the consultant's report), although this problem diminished over time to the point that all records were complete for Macedonia. Follow-up information on patients was not available, nor were comparisons possible with patients seen at the deployed hospital. In addition, there were no data on patient or provider satisfaction, response time, or costs. The majority of consults were for acute problems that were not emergencies, and the most frequent questions involved recommendations for further treatment. Dermatology was the specialty most often consulted (suggesting that perhaps dermatologists ought to be routinely deployed). Reviews of records by experts suggested that the consultation significantly changed the diagnosis in 30 percent of the cases and significantly changed the treatment in 32 percent of the cases. Change was more likely for seriously ill patients. The expert reviewers concluded that the consult was essential or prevented evacuation in about 10 percent of the cases and was not needed in an equal percentage; it was helpful or significantly helpful in the majority of the other cases. Consults dropped off after deployed physicians familiar with the program were rotated out.

This study highlighted issues identified in other studies. One was the problem of sustaining telemedicine consultations over time because the initial group of trained participants left, because the technology was awkward, or because participants at distant sites learned enough during initial consultations to handle subsequent patients. It also demonstrated the difficulty of conducting prospective studies and, even with retrospective studies, of tracking patient outcomes. The "difference in diagnosis" variable and expert judgments were used because data on differences in health outcomes were unavailable or too costly to collect.

Research Under Way on
Teledermatology Services for Rural Areas

As mentioned above, dermatology has proven to be a major generator of telemedicine consultations. One project at the Oregon Health Sciences University (OHSU) was described above. Researchers there are also testing dermatology consultation services in rural sites over a two-year period. The project will test "whether this technology will improve the process of health care delivery by increasing information flow and reducing isolation; improving the provision of dermatologic care; and increasing the primary care provider's knowledge of dermatology" (Perednia and Brown, 1995, p. 46). The project is also designed to develop an application with the potential to sustain itself once federal funding ceases. It relies on ordinary phone service and off-the-shelf equipment that, although not necessarily shareable for other telemedicine applications, is inexpensive to operate.

The experiences of the project investigators illustrate the difficulties of conducting research in distance medicine. For example, attracting and maintaining multiple remote research sites has been difficult. Involvement may depend on personal links (e.g., between a rural physician and the university from which he or she graduated) that may disappear (or at least be interrupted) with retirements or similar events. Phone companies have not been eager to extend improved telecommunications technologies to rural areas, where even basic phone service is sometimes hard to obtain.[5] Competition and other financial pressures are leading health care providers to reduce funding of continuing medical education for staff and withdraw from participation in the telecommunications network that was also to be used for telemedicine.

Three Research Initiatives on Effectiveness and Cost-Effectiveness

The committee discovered several research projects that were intended to apply more rigorous methods to the evaluation of telemedicine and to extend the focus beyond description and feasibility assessments to effectiveness and cost-effectiveness. The three described below illustrate different strategies.

In addition to its other contracts with CHPR, HCFA has also

---

[5]The recent federal telecommunications legislation is intended to reduce the rate disparity between urban and rural areas and thereby improve rural access to these technologies. This will create a subsidy that should be acknowledged in evaluations of telemedicine. Allocating part of the subsidy to telemedicine applications versus other uses (e.g., education, business, personal) would likely be difficult.

contracted with the center to evaluate the medical effectiveness and cost-effectiveness of telemedicine for routine consultative services, medical-surgical follow-up, and management of chronic illness. The study will involve all HCFA telemedicine demonstration sites and, as needed, other sites that are able to participate (up to a total of 15 programs).[6] Patients who receive telemedicine services will be compared with those receiving conventional consultations in a set of comparable control facilities. The goal is to accumulate a total of 2,400 cases (half telemedicine patients and half a comparison group matched insofar as possible for clinical and demographic characteristics).

In conjunction with the Clinical Telemedicine Cooperative Group (CTCG, above), CHPR will develop computerized data collection instruments focused on episodes of care over a nine-month period. The plan is to collect data on (a) fixed and variable program costs; (b) use of services by participating patients; (c) patient demographic characteristics and clinical history; (d) presenting symptoms and complaints; (e) health status; (f) symptom distress; (g) functional capacity; (h) symptom resolution; and (i) characteristics of the consultation. Information collection will involve abstraction of information from patient records, telephone interviews with patients, Medicare records, and other sources.

In a second, experimental phase of the study, CHPR will randomly assign patients to one of four interventions: telephone consultation only; still images with audio or text; interactive video; and face-to-face consultation. The objective is to compare the effectiveness of the alternatives and to identify the marginal effects and costs of each of the additions of information (e.g., shifting from audio only to audio plus still images).

In another HCFA funded project, researchers at the University of Michigan have been collaborating with researchers at the Medical College of Georgia on a project that is intended to both develop a model research methodology and implement it using sites in Georgia and West Virginia (Sanders and Bashshur, 1995). The components of the model (which is a kind of evaluation framework) include the

---

[6]The medical-surgical follow-up component may be dropped based on difficulties in identifying and interviewing control patients within the project schedule (Grigsby, March 7, 1996, letter).

research question, the research design, the data collection instruments, and the data analysis plan. The proposal emphasizes the need to consider not just individual applications or technologies but the system of care in which they are embedded. The research hypothesis stated that telemedicine would improve access, enhance the quality of care, and contain costs. To investigate this hypothesis, the project devised a matrix that included both client and provider perspectives on each of these outcome areas.

The design also draws from educational evaluations the concepts of formative and summative evaluations (Bashshur et al., 1975; Bashshur, 1995; see also Weiss, 1972; and Rutman, 1980). *Formative* evaluations are primarily descriptive, focus on immediate or short-term outcomes, and attempt to identify operational problems, including departures from the program as originally designed. They often emphasize what some call the proof or test of concept (referred to above), that is, the basic operational feasibility of an application with which users have little relevant experience. In contrast, *summative* evaluations tend to focus on programs or applications that are better established. They attempt to discern longer-term effects (including unanticipated or unwanted effects) and provide an overall assessment of whether the program achieved its objectives.

Although these concepts usually are employed to describe different stages in the evolution of research on a topic, this design incorporates both formative and summative aspects. Thus, one phase of research emphasizes the importance of descriptive information on the program's structure (hardware, software, staffing, support systems), the problems encountered, and efforts to resolve them. The other phase originally provided for a quasi-experimental study of clients and providers in two experimental and two control sites and an additional case-control study of episodes of care with and without telemedicine.

As the project has developed further, the methodology has shifted to reflect practical difficulties in implementing the project and in response to requests from the HCFA, the primary funder. The emphasis in West Virginia is on Medicare and financing issues. In addition to an empirical analysis of cost, quality, and access for Medicare inpatients, the project will use a dynamic simulation model to estimate effects in more detail using existing data, expert clinical opinions, and theoretical assumptions. The primary theoretical component for the financial analysis draws on "real options" analysis and operations theory. Real options analysis is designed for situations in which the size and timing of future cash flows is highly uncertain (as is often true for telemedicine) and the use of conventional net-present-value analysis is less applicable (Trigeorgis, 1995).

In a third study funded primarily by the Office of Rural Health Policy, the University of Washington (as part of its involvement in the multistate WAMI—Washington, Alaska, Montana, and Idaho—consortium) has developed a demonstration project involving diverse rural sites and a university-based specialty consultation network. It employs a multisite pretest, posttest research design to assess the feasibility, acceptability, and cost-effectiveness of a telemedicine network (WAMI, unpublished project description, 1995).

As this report was being drafted, the project was in the pretest data collection stage in four quite different sites (ranging from a 22-person physician group to a site staffed by two physicians and a physician assistant). Researchers were preparing an inventory of existing telemedicine links and on-site specialty consultations (by out-of-area practitioners). They were also developing comparative cost information for on-site consultations. The included specialties are radiology, cardiology, dermatology, mental health, obstetrics/paranatology, orthopedics, pediatrics, emergency/trauma care, and neurosurgery. Baseline provider and administrator survey data have been collected.

This project illustrates some of the practical tools that may be used to determine whether the project was implemented as planned and to identify problems that arose during implementation. Remote site participants were to keep detailed logs to capture mostly qualitative data about the various steps involved in putting the telemedicine system into place. In addition, encounter forms were to be generated for every telemedicine contact to track information about the patient, provider, clinical problem, process of care, costs (including grant costs, patient or provider expenses, and in-kind contributions) and difficulties experienced with the equipment or other aspects of the consultation. The project researchers would periodically reinventory telemedicine linkages to track changes, survey patient and provider satisfaction, and collect general comments about user experience. Researchers stated that they would try to develop data collection instruments identical or comparable to those of the Clinical

Telemedicine Cooperative Group described earlier (see earlier section on the Telemedicine Research Center).

CONCLUSION

For the series of early demonstration projects funded in the 1970s, the awkward equipment, feasibility oriented projects, small numbers of patients, and high cost per patient served discouraged a sustained program of systematic development and research in telemedicine and apparently contributed to the disappearance of most of these projects. In the late 1980s and 1990s, as the technological base advanced and became more practical to use and as support for outcomes research and clinical evaluations gathered momentum, demonstration projects blossomed once again. The committee's discussions with those now involved in telemedicine evaluations suggest that they continue to face problems of small numbers of cases. In addition, securing relevant and comparable evaluation sites can be difficult given special data collection requirements, differing organizational and professional priorities, and reimbursement limits.

The committee was encouraged by the increased attention to evaluation by government agencies, health care organizations, and researchers and by efforts to develop creative strategies for overcoming or compensating for difficulties in undertaking sound evaluations. This work provides an important starting point. Much, however, remains to be done to build evaluation into telemedicine programs and to see more well-designed and well-executed studies of specific applications carried to conclusion. The next chapter presents the committee's framework for such studies.

6

A Framework for Planning and
Improving Evaluations of Telemedicine

In some respects, telemedicine is still a frontier. Rigorous evaluative discipline can be difficult to apply amidst the effort and enthusiasm that comes with developing projects, coping with immature technologies, gaining financial or political support, or building new markets. Systematic evaluations require time to plan, fund, and implement, and the evaluation projects inspired by the recent resurgence of interest in telemedicine generally have yet to be completed and reported. As a result, the models and information available to the committee were limited, although the committee learned much from the work that has been done.

Continued improvement in the field will depend on agreement by those interested in telemedicine that it is important to invest in systematic evaluation of telemedicine's effects on the quality, accessibility, cost, and acceptability of health care. The evaluation framework presented in this chapter attempts to relate broadly accepted strategies of health services research and evaluation research in general to some of the challenges and problems in evaluating telemedicine that have been described in preceding chapters.

Starting with the general principles set forth in Chapter 1, the committee devised several principles more specific to the task of developing the evaluation framework for clinical applications of telemedicine. First, evaluation should be viewed as an integral part of program design, implementation, and redesign. Second, evaluation should be understood as a cumulative and forward-looking process for building useful knowledge and as guidance for program or policy improvement rather than as an isolated exercise in project assessment. Third, the benefits and costs of specific telemedicine applications should be compared with those of current practice or reasonable alternatives to current practice. Careful comparison is the core of evaluation.

Fourth, the potential benefits and costs of telemedicine should be broadly construed to promote the identification and measurement of unexpected and possibly unwanted effects and to encourage an assessment of overall effects on all significant parties. Fifth, in considering evaluation options and strategies, the accent should be on identifying the least costly and most practical ways of achieving desired results rather than investigating the most exciting or advanced telemedicine options. Sixth, by focusing on the clinical, financial, institutional, and social objectives and needs of those who may benefit or suffer from telemedicine, evaluations can avoid excessive preoccupation with the characteristics and demands of individual technologies.

The committee recognizes that actual evaluations face a variety of methodological, financial, political, and organizational constraints. Nonetheless, based on its review of current applications and evaluations, the committee believes that considerable improvement can be achieved in the quality and rigor of telemedicine evaluations and, thereby, in the utility of the information and guidance they provide to decisionmakers.

PLANNING FOR EVALUATION

Before presenting the evaluation framework, the committee thought it was important to underscore the significance of systematic planning for evaluation. Evaluation is too often an afterthought, considered after the seemingly more important issues of putting a program together are settled. This approach jeopardizes the potential for the evaluation plan, the program plan, and program implementation to operate together to answer questions about the program's benefits and costs. For example, an effort to assess whether a telemedicine application is likely to be sustainable after a demonstration period will be more useful if the conditions for sustained operation are considered in planning the personnel, procedures, organizational linkages, outcomes and financial data, and other aspects of the test application. Although evaluation strategies must necessarily be tailored to fit the policy or management concerns and the characteristics of different fields (e.g., education, public safety, health care), certain questions, concepts, and steps are common to the planning of successful evaluations. They include

- establishing evaluation objectives;
- setting priorities for the selection of specific applications to be evaluated;
- assessing the probable feasibility of an evaluation, including the availability of adequate funding and the likelihood of adequate cooperation from relevant parties;
- identifying the particular intervention to be evaluated, the alternatives to which it will be compared, the outcomes of interest, and the level and timing of evaluation;
- specifying the expected relationships between interventions and outcomes and the other factors that might affect these relationships; and
- developing an evaluation strategy that includes a credible and feasible research design and analysis plan.

This list reflects several decades' worth of work in many disciplines to create scientifically respectable evaluation strategies that are also useful to decisionmakers and feasible to implement (see, e.g., Suchman, 1967; Weiss, 1972; NAS, 1978; Cook and Campbell, 1979; Sechrest, 1979; OTA, 1980a; Rutman, 1980; Wortman, 1981; Tufte, 1983, 1990; Rossi and Freeman, 1989; Mohr, 1988; Flagle, 1990; Wholey et al., 1994). Although this report was not intended to be a how-to-do-it manual, or to duplicate existing texts, the discussion below briefly discusses the above steps. Readers should, however, consult the references cited above—as well as those cited below and in the preceding chapter—for more detailed guidance.

Establishing Evaluation Objectives

Ideally, evaluation needs will be considered in the early stages of planning for pilot programs. This implies the identification of clear objectives for the program, the stipulation of results that would indicate whether the program has met its objectives, and the specification of steps to collect relevant data about the program's operations and effects.

Several important questions will ordinarily be considered in establishing the objectives for a particular evaluation. They include: What kinds of decisions may be affected by the results? Who will be the primary users of evaluation results? Who is sponsoring the evaluation and why? Who else has a major stake in the evaluation results?

Determining the objectives—and, thus, the important questions to be answered or concerns to be addressed—for a particular evaluation may not be completely straightforward. In some cases, programs and activities evolve incrementally without much attention to well-argued rationales. Moreover, stated rationales may not always capture program goals, perhaps because the goals have not been carefully thought through or perhaps because underlying motivations are somewhat different from those that are declared. The latter situation may require that study designs be sensitive to political currents. In any case, investigators should seek to determine either what their target program was originally intended to accomplish or what objectives it may serve in the current environment (regardless of the past) or both.

Even if program objectives are relatively clear, other considerations such as evaluation feasibility and anticipated concerns of possible future funders may influence the choice of specific evaluation questions. Government agencies, private foundations, and vendors will usually have interests related to public policies or market strategies that go beyond those of specific demonstration sites. Although project objectives can sometimes be stated in some order of priority, how they will be balanced and what trade-offs will have to be considered may be difficult to specify precisely in advance.

The varying interests of project and evaluation sponsors are reflected in the expectations for the telemedicine projects supported by different federal agencies. For example, the Office of Rural Health Policy focuses on quality, accessibility, and cost of health care in rural areas. Although the Health Care Financing Administration is also interested in quality and access, its sponsored projects are intended primarily to provide information that will help the agency formulate payment policies for Medicare. These differences in interest notwithstanding, federal agencies have been working together (as described in the preceding chapter) to formulate an umbrella framework for project evaluation that is intended to make it easier to aggregate conclusions from individual evaluations.

Setting Priorities

As is true for any activity, resources for evaluating telemedicine applications are limited, and funding for an evaluation may compete with funding for the services to be evaluated. Making the case for research to distinguish what works from what does not is easier in theory than in practice, for example, in cases when decisions have to be made between funding patient care at higher levels or funding program evaluation.

Those sponsoring or conducting evaluations generally have to consider priorities for the use of limited resources in making two kinds of decisions: selection of topics and selection of evaluation strategies or methods. Topic selection is often handled quite informally, but a more formal or explicit process of setting priorities may help decisionmakers focus limited resources more rationally. Several core questions are generally relevant to any priority-setting exercise (IOM, 1992b, 1995b). These questions, which are framed below in terms of possible clinical applications of telemedicine, include

- How common is the telemedicine application now? How common is it likely to be?
  - How significant is the problem addressed by the application?
    — prevalence of the problem
    — burden of illness (e.g., mortality, quality of life)
    — cost of managing the problem
    — variability across regions or population subgroups
- What is the likelihood that evaluation results will affect decisions about adoption of the application, its integration into routine operations, and other missions of the venture?
- Will the study wastefully duplicate or constructively supplement conclusions from other evaluations?

Most of these considerations assume a societal or policy-level perspective. They are most likely to be raised by organizations such as the Department of Defense, the National Library of Medicine, and the Office of Rural Health Policy that fund a variety of telemedicine projects and have a formal commitment to program evaluation. Nonetheless, health plans, health care delivery organizations, and vendors of communications and information technologies may also consider similar questions in determining where they will direct resources for systematic analysis and evaluation.

The resource issues in selecting a research design revolve around three basic questions. First, what are the costs associated with different research strategies? Second, what are the costs of a strategy relative to its potential to provide answers to the evaluation questions? Third, is the cost of the evaluation strategy reasonable in relation to the potential costs and benefits of the application or program to be evaluated?

In practice, evaluations often follow targets of opportunity. That is, they are designed to take advantage of the programs or capacities of an established institution or the political appeal of certain topics. For example, if a medical center has an energetic and determined specialist willing and able to design an application and secure funds, that person's project may take priority over applications with (theoretically) more organizational relevance. Likewise, if demonstration funds are confined to projects involving rural areas, urban applications with more potential benefit may be neglected.

Determining the Feasibility of Evaluation

In addition to costs, a number of other factors may affect the feasibility of an evaluation. Some factors have behavioral or political aspects. These include whether those responsible for the application or program in question will cooperate and whether the intended beneficiaries of a program will agree to provide the information needed from them. A different but possibly relevant question is whether the intended audience for the evaluation will be receptive to results that may run counter to their preferences or self-interest.

Other considerations are quite practical. Will the needed information be available on a timely basis? If not, what steps would need to be taken to provide it, and how long would it take to implement those steps? Are the time demands for information collection excessive for program staff or beneficiaries?

Another practical issue involves the timing of an evaluation. Because most evaluations look for effects within a relatively short period of a few months or perhaps two to three years, timing can be a problem if the key results emerge over a longer term and if short-term outcomes are not good proxies for these long-term results. Moreover, evaluating a program before start-up problems are resolved may produce misleading results. Evaluating a program too late may also lead to problems if, for example, users are so comfortable with an intervention that they will not agree to be part of a control group not subject to the intervention.

Feasibility assessments are also relevant to decisions about the alternatives to which the telemedicine application will be compared. If the preferred comparison sites will not or cannot participate, the comparison group may have to be the experimental group before the telemedicine application is initiated or after it has been concluded. This kind of before-and-after single group design is a relatively weak evaluation strategy, although measures taken at multiple points before, during, or after the telemedicine test will strengthen the design (see, e.g., Cook and Campbell, 1979).

The choice of appropriate comparisons will depend, in part, on whether the application is in the earlier or later stages of development. For example, when image quality is yet to be established, an evaluation may compare diagnoses based on digital images with diagnoses based on conventional film-based images or direct patient examination. The next stage would extend the evaluative focus to consider other issues of quality, access, cost, patient and clinician acceptance, and feasibility in real practice settings. For example, in a project described in Chapter 5, physicians in one set of rural practices would be able to consult on dermatology problems via telemedicine while physicians in another set of practices would continue their traditional referral patterns. In some cases, the alternative might be doing nothing, but only if that is what would be expected in the absence of a program.

Although general methodological and statistical principles exist to guide a multiplicity of evaluation tasks, no "one size fits all" evaluation plan exists. For example, if an evaluation is an early "test of concept" to determine the basic technical and procedural feasibility of a telemedicine application (e.g., home health monitoring), the research design and measures will likely differ from a later project intended to help decisionmakers decide whether the application should be adopted as a regular service of a health care organization.

ELEMENTS OF AN EVALUATION

The committee identified several basic elements that should be considered in planning and reporting an evaluation, whether that evaluation is very tightly focused or broader in scope. These elements include

- Project description and research question(s)
- Strategic objectives
- Clinical objectives
- Business plan or project management plan
- Level and perspective of evaluation
- Research design and analysis plan
  — characteristics of experimental and comparison groups
  — technical, clinical, and administrative processes
  — measurable outcomes
  — sensitivity analysis
- Documentation of methods and results

Although these elements are necessarily described individually and sequentially below, the development of an evaluation plan involves the continuing interplay and rethinking of elements as their conceptual and practical implications are assessed and reassessed. Moreover, during implementation, evaluators often find they need to revise the evaluation plan. In sum, the process of planning and implementing an evaluation flows logically but not always in a strictly linear fashion.

Project Description and Research Questions

The *project description* identifies the application that is being evaluated and the alternative(s) to which it is being compared. For example, the application might be described concisely as a dermatology consultation program using a one-way video and two-way audio link between a consulting center and two rural primary care sites. Two other rural sites would maintain their existing consulting practices. A thorough program description would more precisely and completely identify the characteristics of the telemedicine and comparison services including relevant hardware and software employed, restrictions on the clinical problems or patients to be studied, the length of the project, and the project personnel.

Specifying the basic *research question* or questions—the hypothesized link between the program intervention and desired outcomes—is a critical evaluation step. It encourages systematic thinking about how program interventions are expected to affect the outcomes of interest; what other factors may influence that link; and which different research designs and measurement strategies best fit the problem.

By identifying the expected intermediate changes that an intervention must set in motion if the desired outcome is to occur, evaluators will be in a better position to give decisionmakers useful information on what contributed to a program's success or failure. For example, research on programs designed to change personal health habits or physician practice patterns have made it clear that not only must a service or decision guide be available, it must also be accepted and adopted (Avorn and Soumerai, 1983; Eisenberg, 1986; Soumerai and Avorn, 1990; Green, 1991; IOM, 1992a; Kaluzny et al., 1995). This research implies that potential clinician users of telemedicine, for instance, must (a) know an option is available; (b) understand the minimum details necessary to use it; (c) accept it, that is, conclude that its potential advantages (e.g., better clinical information or better patient access to care) outweigh its apparent disadvantages (e.g., inconvenient scheduling); and (d) act on the basis of their knowledge and conclusions. If one or more of these intermediate events fail to occur for all or most of the clinicians involved, then an application is likely to fail.

Strategic and Clinical Objectives

The *strategic objectives* in an evaluation plan state how the telemedicine project is intended to affect the organization's or sponsor's goals and how the evaluation strategy relates to those objectives. These goals might include improving health services in rural areas, keeping deployed soldiers in the field, reducing expenses for government-funded medical care, or strengthening an organization's competitive position. Competitive position is broadly construed to extend beyond the marketplace to encompass the need of public organizations to demonstrate their value to the policymakers who determine which programs will survive in an era of government retrenchment and health care cost containment. For instance, the early strategic objectives for a telemedicine program at an academic medical center might be to add to the telemedicine knowledge base (and thereby serve the institution's research mission) and to establish or strengthen the center's research reputation in the field (and thereby lay the base for future funding). Depending on the results, later strategic objectives might relate more to the patient care mission or to reinforcing the institution's position in local, regional, and broader health care markets.

The *clinical objectives* state how the telemedicine project is intended to affect individual or population health by changing the quality, accessibility, or cost of care. For example, a project might be intended to allow more frequent, economical, and convenient monitoring of homebound patients than is provided by existing home and office visit arrangements or it might be designed to improve access to appropriate specialty services for a rural population.

To the extent possible, evaluators should identify *in advance* what constitutes favorable or unfavorable outcomes in a particular context. For example, does a clinical application of telemedicine need to show performance better than, equivalent to, or almost as good as the alternative(s) to which it is being compared? Depending on the outcome at issue, the goals of the project sponsor, and other factors such as severe cost constraints, the answer may vary. Thus, if an application was expected to (and did) substantially reduce costs and if costs were thought to be the dominant issue for the organization's customers, then an organization might consider a slight decrease in patient satisfaction to be tolerable. Although the judgment of the outcome or the way different outcomes are balanced may vary depending on the perspective, the definition, measurement, or calculation of the outcome should not differ.

Level and Perspective of Evaluation

Once the research questions and objectives have been established, the appropriate level and perspective of an evaluation will usually become apparent. Although they may overlap to some degree, at least three broad levels can be distinguished: clinical, institutional, and societal. Somewhat different evaluation strategies may be appropriate for various levels of decisionmaking.

At the *clinical* level, the evaluative focus is on the benefits, risks, and costs of alternative approaches to a health problem. For example, does digital teleradiology provide clinically acceptable images for breast cancer screening? What are the benefits and harms of telepsychiatry compared to the alternatives? Clinical evaluations provide critical guidance for decisions about individual patient care. An institutional decision to adopt a technology will, however, ordinarily require additional evidence of its feasibility and value.

At the *institutional* level, the focus includes not only the application but also its organizational context including administrative structures and practices, clients or customers, clinical and other personnel, and clinical protocols. An institution-level evaluation might ask the following kinds of questions: Has a teleradiology link between a rural hospital and an urban radiology center affected referrals or revenues for each institution? Does a telemedicine link for troops in remote locations reduce medical evacuations? Are clinicians and patients at each site satisfied with a teledermatology link between a university medical center and a capitated medical group? How do the costs compare to the alternatives (e.g., physically referring patients, adding another dermatologist to the group)? What factors (e.g., equipment location or ease of use) appear to underlie the results (positive or negative)? Positive results at this stage of evaluation may encourage diffusion of a technology on an institution-by-institution basis.

At the *system* or *societal* level, the focus expands to incorporate broader health care delivery and financing issues, particularly those involving the allocation of public resources. For example, does telemedicine have a role to play in state policies to support rural medical services? Or, more specifically, how do particular telemedicine applications compare to other policy options, such as area health education centers, direct subsidies for rural hospitals, and educational loan programs linked to practice in underserved areas? If the evaluation results look positive at this level, decisionmakers may support broad adoption and diffusion of the technology.

In developing an evaluative framework and related criteria, this committee has attempted to keep in mind evaluation issues at each of these levels. The distinctions are particularly relevant in the areas of quality and cost because conclusions about the merits of a particular application of telemedicine may differ depending on whether one considers individual, institutional, or societal interests. Moreover, the committee recognized that, depending on the sponsor and audience, program-level and system-level questions may be both intertwined and overlooked. For example, telemedicine may save patients money by eliminating transportation and accommodations expenses for travel to a distant consultant. Evaluations driven by purchaser (e.g., insurer) or supplier (e.g., hospital) concerns may or may not consider such savings.

Business or Project Management Plan

The committee concluded that a significant weakness of many demonstration projects and their evaluations has been the lack of a business plan that sets forth how the implementation and evaluation of the project are designed to provide information that decision-makers can use to decide whether the test application is financially sustainable as an ongoing program. It is likely that the demise of many telemedicine programs can be attributed to an incomplete understanding of the business case for establishing and maintaining a telemedicine program and an inadequate appreciation of the costs involved.

In some cases, the business plan may be little more than the *project management plan* for an early exploration (test of concept) of a telemedicine application. That is, it will outline the project's leadership and management structures, its work plan and schedule, and its budget. In other cases, the *business plan* will be much more extensive, incorporating a detailed financial analysis and an appraisal of the program's fit with the organization's strategic plan.

On the financial side, a formal business plan typically would include start-up and operating budgets for the project, a break-even analysis, income projections (a profit and loss statement), and cash flow projections. Although details will vary depending on the type of project, its sponsor, its tax status (e.g., not-for-profit), and other factors, a start-up budget should allow for the following expenses prior to the time the project becomes operational: personnel costs prior to opening; consultant fees; travel; equipment and supplies; salaries and wages; insurance; utilities; and any overhead or other charges that may be required by the parent organization. An operating budget should include money to cover expenses for the first three to six months of operation and would, for most evaluations, include many of the same kinds of expenses (e.g., salaries, supplies) included in the start-up budget.

If it is clear that the project is being evaluated as a possible component of its parent organization's overall business plan, then the project business plan usually would include a multiyear summary of the income statement and cash flow projections, with more detailed monthly projections for the first year and quarterly projections for later years. Each should be backed by documentation of assumptions, for example, about revenue sources.

Research Design and Analysis Plan

The *research design* describes the strategy and steps for developing valid comparative information, including the sources and techniques for collecting data. It specifies whether the strategy is experimental, quasi-experimental, or nonexperimental and presents the rationale and the limitations of the approach. The *analysis plan* outlines the methods for analyzing and interpreting the resulting information. Depending on the nature of the information collected and the research design, these methods may range from relatively simple tabular comparisons to sophisticated multivariate regression analyses.

Initiatives to evaluate education, welfare, criminal justice, public health, and other nonclinical programs have generated a large literature on evaluation research designs (see, e.g., Campbell and Stanley, 1963; Suchman, 1967; Weiss, 1972; Cook and Campbell, 1979; Sechrest, 1979; Rossi et al., 1983; Fink, 1993; Wholey et al., 1994). This literature provides systematic assessments of the strengths and limitations of different research designs (see the addendum to this chapter for further discussion). It also describes and encourages creative attempts to minimize or correct some of the limitations of the weaker but more feasible designs.

Much of the program evaluation literature suggests, to paraphrase an old saying, that "it is better to be roughly right than to be precisely ignorant" (Wholey et al., 1994, p. 1). This should not be taken as an excuse for a sloppy evaluation, but the rigor of the research design may reasonably depend on how much experience has accumulated with the intervention or program being evaluated and the uses that will be made of findings. Overall, the basic challenge in research design is to balance the need for confidence in the findings of research with the demand for relevance, feasibility, and afford-ability. Trust in the findings of research hinges primarily on judg-ments about internal and external validity (see addendum) and about an evaluator's freedom from serious bias or conflict of interest.

Characteristics of Experimental and Comparison Groups

The research design specifies the experimental group or groups that will be provided telemedicine services and the comparison (or control) group or groups that will be provided alternative services. Except perhaps in the early "test of concept" stage, when the assess-ment focuses on whether an application can even be implemented, comparison is central to evaluation. Unfortunately, as suggested earlier, telemedicine evaluators may find it very difficult to recruit appropriate comparison groups, especially when there is no organi-zational or financial incentive for participation.

Typically, evaluators will want to describe carefully a number of characteristics of experimental and control groups that might affect outcomes and complicate conclusions about the effect of the experi-mental intervention. The starting point for identifying such charac-teristics is the basic research question for the project, which will suggest a series of additional questions—drawn from past research, judgment, and experience—about other independent factors or vari-ables that may intensify, block, or confound the relationship be-tween the experimental and dependent variables. These factors usu-ally include but are not limited to

- patient characteristics (e.g., age, sex, race, severity of illness);
- provider characteristics and relationships (e.g., nurse practi-tioners, salaried primary care physicians);
- organizational characteristics and linkages (e.g., independent primary care practice, unit of an integrated health system);
- financial and legal environment (e.g., sources of revenues, regulatory restrictions); and
- geographic setting (e.g., urban or rural).

To identify the effect of the telemedicine application on the de-pendent variables or outcomes, these other factors should be "controlled" through the research design or statistical methods. As briefly described in the addendum to this chapter, random assignment of patients to experimental and control groups is a classic method (actually, a variety of methods) to control for differences in patient characteristics. Often, however, researchers must rely on statistical or other techniques for controlling for differences. For example, to control for (rather than to determine) the effect of different provider payment methods, an evaluation might be restricted to either capitated or fee-for-service sites; alternatively, payment method might be used as a control variable in a multivariate statistical analysis.

Technical, Clinical, and Administrative Processes

In defining the application and comparison services to be evaluated and identifying the objectives of the evaluation, many elements of the project's clinical, technical, and administrative processes will become evident. The *technical infrastructure* includes not only the immediate hardware and software requirements of the application but also the larger information and communications systems available to support them (as described in Chapter 3). For example, if a project links an urban medical center and a rural clinic, what personnel are available to assist each site with technical problems? If the system depends on a satellite link, what scheduling and other restrictions apply? Will information about patients be available from a computer-based patient record or will the information have to be specially entered and collected for the project?

Clinical processes are the way medical services are to be provided as part of the telemedicine project. Often, they are precisely set forth in a clinical protocol that identifies specific activities, their order and timing, responsible personnel, circumstances that trigger different protocols, and appropriate clinical documentation. Like technical processes, these processes are supported by a larger clinical care system that includes, for example, procedures for maintaining medical equipment, distributing medications, scheduling work flow, and monitoring clinical performance.

Administrative processes also include any array of financial, legal, personnel, security, and facilities management. The most immediately relevant of these (e.g., procedures for establishing new staff positions, hiring personnel, purchasing equipment and services, receiving funds, paying bills, and referring patients) will ordinarily be identified as part of program and evaluation planning.

In addition to describing technical, clinical, and administrative processes as they are expected to operate and establishing steps to implement these processes, evaluators need to track processes *as they actually occur* to identify shortfalls and unanticipated problems or complications. If, for example, a homebound patient is to demonstrate range of motion in front of a camera, an evaluation should document whether patients follow the instructions well enough for the distant clinician to make an assessment. To cite another case, if military clinicians try to use telemedicine services but find that the clinical protocols are irritating, the equipment does not work, or the consultants are not scheduled appropriately, an evaluation needs to document this and, if possible, suggest how the problem could be resolved. Event or problem logs kept by project personnel may be used to record (for later analysis) departures from planned processes as well as unexpected events and problems.

Without efforts to implement interventions as planned and to monitor the extent to which this happens, evaluators will find it difficult to distinguish between a failure of the telemedicine application and a failure to implement the application as intended. Such distinctions are critically important to those making decisions about whether to adopt, substantially redesign, or discontinue telemedicine programs.

Measurable Outcomes

Measurable outcomes identify the variables and the data to be collected to determine whether the project is meeting its clinical and strategic objectives. This committee was asked to focus on issues in evaluating quality, access, and costs for clinical applications of telemedicine. It also concluded that the acceptability of telemedicine to patients and clinicians warranted separate attention, although patient satisfaction frequently figures in assessments of quality of care, access, and cost-effectiveness. Depending on its objectives, an evaluation may consider a range of other outcomes related to an organization's competitive position, its relationships with other institutions, the demand for different kinds of health care personnel, the economic health of a community, or other effects.

In addition to outcomes desired from the project, decisionmakers will also benefit from evaluations that attempt to identify and measure possible unwanted and unexpected outcomes. A case in point is the "training effect" that appears to operate in some telemedicine programs such that the distant clinicians who participate in telemedicine consultations learn enough about diagnosis and patient management that they no longer need telemedicine consultations when they encounter certain patient problems. The benefit of such clinician education, however, may create a dilemma if demand for telemedicine consultations drops too low to justify continuation of a program. How such results might factor into decisions about the future of an application is not clear, but it would undoubtedly affect the interpretation of utilization statistics.

The specification of outcomes to be measured should describe the time frame for the measurements, for example, rehospitalization within six months of discharge or patient satisfaction with telemedicine at the time of service. One of the most frequent limitations of clinical and program evaluations is their focus on relatively short-term outcomes. This focus is borne of time and budget constraints and data collection difficulties. These difficulties are especially acute for longer-term health and cost outcomes. Depending on the objectives, circumstances, and resources, an evaluation may involve a range of immediate, intermediate, and long-term outcome measures, as discussed further in Chapter 7.

Sensitivity Analysis

Because the committee believed that the fast pace of change and other uncertainties surrounding telemedicine applications were particular challenges, it highlighted one element of an analysis plan—sensitivity analyses—as a distinct item in the evaluation framework. *Sensitivity analyses* explore the extent to which conclusions may change if values of key variables or assumptions change. For example, financial projections may show the impact of different assumptions about costs for purchasing and maintaining telecommunications and other equipment. As noted above, a particular problem for telemedicine evaluations is the stability of technology or environment. With data capture, transmission, and display technologies improving in quality and declining in cost, evaluators may need to consider (a) how sensitive their conclusions may be to technological change and (b) how analyses might be constructed to estimate the impact of certain kinds of changes. For example, an analysis of cost-effectiveness could include a sensitivity analysis that incorporates different assumptions about the timing and cost of key hardware or software upgrades or replacement (Briggs et al., 1994; Hamby, 1995).

Documentation of Methods and Results

In reviewing evaluations of telemedicine applications, the committee was often frustrated by the incomplete or casual documentation of the methods employed and the specific findings. One result was to diminish the utility and credibility of the reports. Efforts to identify weaknesses and improve documentation in research reports have been undertaken by a number of medical and health services research journals, including the *Journal of the American Medical Association, Annals of Internal Medicine, Health Services Research,* and *Medical Care.* They have developed guidelines and procedures to improve the clarity and specificity of abstracts, the processes of peer review, and the reporting of methods (including randomization procedures, sample sizes, and statistical power), data analysis and reporting, and sponsorship. (See, for example, DerSimonian et al., 1982; Pocock et al., 1987; Haynes et al., 1990; Altman and Goodman, 1994; Moher et al., 1994; Schulz et al., 1994; Sweitzer and Cullen, 1994; Taddio et al., 1994; Rennie, 1995; and Schulz, 1995.) At least one telemedicine publication, *Telemedicine Journal,* is attempting to follow this guidance. Although these suggestions have been aimed at journal editors, they have the important additional benefit of reinforcing basic principles of sound research and statistical analysis.

EVALUATION AND CONTINUOUS IMPROVEMENT

As noted at the beginning of this chapter, one objective of evaluation and applied research generally is to provide decisionmakers with information that will help them redesign and improve programs. This is particularly true for evaluations conducted in the context of a continuous quality improvement process. The tenets of continuous quality improvement, which were derived in considerable measure from industrial applications, are described in detail elsewhere (see, e.g., Deming, 1986; Batalden and Buchanan, 1989;

Berwick, 1989; Berwick et al., 1990; IOM, 1990c, 1992a; Roberts, 1991; Williamson, 1991; Horn and Hopkins, 1994). Consistent with the evaluation framework set forth here are the principles calling for (a) planning, control, assessment, and improvement activities grounded in statistical and scientific precepts and techniques and (b) standardization of processes to reduce the opportunity for error and to link specific care processes to health outcomes.

Another key principle emphasizes close relationships between customers and suppliers, for example, patients and providers or providers and suppliers of equipment or services. The application of this principle to the design and evaluation of telemedicine applications would address one of the human factor problems identified in Chapter 3: inadequate assessment of and attention to user needs.

The very process of implementing a program and its evaluation components may make evaluators aware of program deficiencies or environmental obstacles to program success. For example, potential participants may balk at using equipment that is inconveniently located or difficult to apply. In addition, the evaluation frameworks and plans reviewed by the committee suggested a number of other means for securing information for program improvement. These included logs kept by clinical or technical personnel and individual or group "debriefing" interviews with participants. These strategies may identify poorly designed or located equipment, "user-unfriendly" software, inadequate training of personnel, bureaucratic burdens, or deficient patient record systems.

Unfortunately, depending on the problems identified, the path to program redesign or improvement may or may not lie within the feasible reach of program administrators or sponsors. For example, some equipment deficiencies may be corrected by switching hardware but others may be resolved only if manufacturers are willing or technically able to fix them.

In general, evaluations based on continuous improvement principles will expect that mistakes or poor outcomes are more often the result of system defects (e.g., poor scheduling systems) than of individual deficiencies. In an environment governed by this outlook, program evaluations may provoke less apprehension and win more cooperation from those whose activities are being studied.

CONCLUSION

Based on its review of current applications and evaluations, the committee concluded that significant improvements are possible in the quality and rigor of telemedicine evaluations. This chapter has emphasized the importance of considering evaluation objectives and strategies during the early stages of program planning. Likewise, it has stressed the value of developing a business plan that explicitly states how the evaluation will provide information to help decision-makers determine whether a telemedicine application is useful, consistent with their strategic plan, and sustainable beyond the initial evaluation stage.

The fast pace of change and other uncertainties surrounding telemedicine applications argue strongly for sensitivity analyses to explore how conclusions may change if values of key variables or assumptions change. It also argues for thinking broadly about potential benefits and costs, carefully documenting how the technical infrastructure and the clinical processes of care were intended to operate, *and* tracking what actually does occur. This latter step is crucial if evaluators who find negative results are to determine, for example, whether the hypothesis linking independent and dependent variables is untenable or whether the hypothesis was not actually tested because the application was not implemented as intended. By tracking what actually happened, evaluators also may achieve a fuller understanding of critical success factors or the factors that, if changed, might improve results.

The evaluation framework presented in this chapter is, in the lexicon of information technologies, a basic evaluation platform that incorporates general evaluation principles, principles adapted to the health care field, and elements of strategies proposed by those encouraging and conducting evaluations of clinical telemedicine. The framework is intended to promote improvements in individual evaluations, but the committee also encourages the coordination of evaluation strategies across projects and organizations, when possible.

ADDENDUM: EXPERIMENTAL, QUASI-EXPERIMENTAL, AND NONEXPERIMENTAL DESIGNS

As noted in the text of Chapter 6, a large literature on evaluation research designs exists to guide those planning evaluations of telemedicine and other activities (see, e.g., Campbell and Stanley, 1963; Suchman, 1967; Weiss, 1972; Cook and Campbell, 1979; Sechrest, 1979; Rossi et al., 1983; Fink, 1993; Wholey et al., 1994). One value of this work is that much of it is not just theoretical but highly practical in its attempts to develop and encourage creative but respectable ways of handling difficult evaluation problems. These efforts revolve around concerns with internal and external validity.

In a 1963 discussion that has become a classic source for evaluation research, Campbell and Stanley set forth an analysis of validity and threats to validity and provided a systematic assessment of the strengths and limitations of various common research designs. Internal validity focuses on the fundamental question: "Did in fact the experimental treatments make a difference in this specific experimental instance?" (Campbell and Stanley, 1963, p. 5). External validity focuses on the extent to which the procedures and results of a particular experiment can be generalized to other populations, settings, and circumstances.

Box 6.1 lists the common threats to internal validity as identified by Campbell and Stanley. It also provides hypothetical illustrations of how they may appear in evaluations of telemedicine applications.

Threats to external validity involve a variety of differences between the groups studied and the groups to which the results might be generalized. For example, generalizing to urban settings from projects in rural areas may be risky. A project that used physicians knowledgeable and enthusiastic about computer-assisted medicine might not produce results applicable to physicians without such knowledge and enthusiasm. A project undertaken in a fee-for-service environment might be less relevant in managed care markets.

In general, research designs can be categorized as experimental, quasi-experimental, or nonexperimental. A true experimental design has two special characteristics. The first is that the design includes at least one group that is subjected to a carefully specified intervention or treatment and another that is subjected to a different intervention. The second characteristic is the random assignment of the subjects (e.g., patients) to the experimental and control groups. Ideally, experimental designs are also "double blinded" in that neither the investigators nor the patients know which group is receiving which treatment.

The most highly structured randomized clinical trials (RCTs) have generally aimed to establish *efficacy* (effects under tightly con-

Box 6.1
Threats to the Internal Validity of Evaluations

1. "History, the specific events occurring between the first and second measurement in addition to the experimental measurement."
Example: During the course of a telepsychiatry project in a poor rural area, a public clinic adds a psychiatric social worker to its staff and thereby makes access to on-site mental health services easier.

2. "Maturation, processes within the respondents [those being studied] operating as a function of the passage of time per se (not specific to the particular events), including growing older, hungrier, more tired, and the like."
Example: In a long-term monitoring program for seriously ill, homebound elderly patients, an unrecognized decrease in functional abilities may limit patients' capacity to carry out instructions successfully, potentially compromising evaluators' ability to assess the program and suggest ways it might be redesigned.

3. "Testing, the effects of taking a test upon the scores of a second testing."
Example: As primary care physicians participate in a series of teleconsultations for a particular clinical problem, they gain sufficient expertise in diagnosis and management that they no longer seek consultations for the problem.

4. "Instrumentation, in which changes in the calibration of a measuring instrument or changes in the observers or scorers used may produce changes in the obtained measurements."
Example: In the midst of a test of digital radiography, a new radiologist, who replaces a more experienced radiologist, takes over the comparison of digitally transmitted images against original films.

5. "Statistical regression [regression to the mean], operating where groups have been selected on the basis of their extreme scores."
Example: Of diabetic patients who have been treated for hypoglycemia, those who test lowest on their understanding of appropriate dietary practices are called weekly by nurses or nutritionists.

6. "Biases resulting in differential *selection* of respondents for the comparison groups."
Example: In a telepsychiatry evaluation that involved telemedicine and control sites, the control sites include patients with greater experience with psychiatric intervention.

7. "Experimental mortality, or differential loss of respondents for the comparison groups."
Example: In a home care evaluation, sicker patients drop out of the comparison group that was not receiving special services.

SOURCE: Quoted material excerpted from Campbell and Stanley, 1963, pp. 5–6.

trolled conditions) rather than *effectiveness* (results under actual conditions of practice). The strength of RCTs is based on the protection of internal validity through the randomization, restrictive patient selection criteria, masking from researchers and patients which patients are receiving which treatments, and strictly controlling the treatment protocols.

A well-designed RCT may still have problems with external validity or generalizability to less controlled practice settings. For example, a recent retrospective analysis of data from two large HMOs on patients who discontinued antihyperlipidemic drugs (drugs to treat high cholesterol) because of adverse effects and therapeutic ineffectiveness suggested that "rates reported in randomized clinical trials may not give an accurate reflection of the tolerability or effectiveness of therapy in the general population" under ordinary conditions (Andrade et al., 1995).

From a practical perspective, traditional, tightly controlled RCTs suffer several handicaps: they tend to be expensive, time-consuming, complex to plan and administer, and ethically or practically unsuitable for some research questions.* Thus, researchers have sought to develop adaptations and alternatives.

One adaptation of the RCT includes "large simple trials" (Zelen, 1993). Large simple trials are simple primarily in that they ask fewer questions than many traditional RCTs. They would still require random assignment but would also rely more on statistical than physical controls of the research setting. Data collection is streamlined. Patients and clinicians anywhere in the United States or elsewhere could participate in a clinical trial if they met defined eligibility criteria and agreed to follow (and document that they followed) specific treatment protocols. Depending on the complexity of the research and treatment protocols, this openness may demand sophisticated and generally expensive programs of training, monitoring, operating assistance, and auditing. In one of its last reports, the Office of Technology Assessment urged those involved with effectiveness research to explore innovative ways to conduct randomized

---

*Among other technologies, drugs are frequent subjects for randomized clinical trials, in large part because the introduction of new drugs requires approval from the Food and Drug Administration based on evidence of safety and efficacy. Some surgical procedures have been the subject of RCTs, but many are introduced without any rigorous evaluation.

clinical trials and incorporate them into ordinary practice (OTA, 1994).

Another option, the clinical practice study or effectiveness trial, generally involves a relatively rigorous form of quasi-experimental research (Horn and Hopkins, 1994; McDonald and Overhage, 1994; Stiell et al., 1994). Quasi-experimental designs cover a variety of strategies that may or may not include a control group or random assignment. Although they are weaker on internal validity, a strength of clinical practice studies or effectiveness trials is that they better represent actual conditions of practice and may be somewhat less expensive and time consuming. They do not insist on homogeneous patient populations that exclude those with comorbidities or complications that may confound analysis of the link between the experimental intervention and patient outcomes. Instead, they measure relevant patient characteristics using severity assessment tools and statistically adjust for differences in experimental and comparison groups. Further, they accommodate departures from rigid treatment protocols by carefully monitoring and measuring actual treatments and then incorporating these data in the statistical analysis. Because this approach does not disqualify large numbers of patients, it is easier to generate the numbers of cases needed for comparisons. Using regression or other statistical techniques, researchers test which process steps are associated with desirable quality, access, or cost outcomes for different kinds of patients.

Although clinical practice studies tend to focus on shorter- rather than longer-term outcomes, the outcomes include effects that are noticeable and important to patients rather than only those that are physiologically measurable through laboratory or other tests. Such studies are often designed to be replicated easily so that they can be undertaken at multiple sites. Sophisticated computer-based patient information systems make it more acceptable to rely—as a "second best" strategy and with appropriate caution—on statistical control techniques rather than randomization and physical control of "confounding" variables.

The objective of such alternatives is *not* to devalue or replace the RCT but to develop additional sources of systematic information on outcomes that will improve on the anecdotal and informal knowledge base that characterizes much of clinical practice (IOM, 1992a; Horn and Hopkins, 1994; OTA, 1994). Some of the telemedicine research projects discussed in Chapter 5 attempt experimental and quasi-experimental research strategies. Even with less demanding designs, tension will exist between the principles of design and the pressures of real-world evaluation.

Another stream of work on alternatives or supplements to the RCT has emphasized nonexperimental research based on the retrospective analysis of large databases that have often been compiled for other purposes (Roos et al., 1982; Moses, 1990; Hannan et al., 1992; NAHDO, 1993). Until telemedicine applications become much more common and routine and are assigned codes to identify them, large databases are unlikely to be useful sources of data on telemedicine applications.

Nonetheless, those looking ahead to more widespread use of telemedicine should consider how routine collection of data about telemedicine may be useful and what would be required to incorporate such data in large data systems. The appeal of these data sources lies in their relative convenience, large numbers of cases, and ease of statistical analysis. Questions or criticisms related to use of large databases for health services research, performance monitoring, and other purposes involve their completeness, accuracy, relevance, and security from authorized access (IOM, 1994b; Maklan et al., 1994; Kuller, 1995). A variety of initiatives have focused on means to reduce the amount of missing data, validate and improve coding of clinical and other information, add information (e.g., death records), and develop methods to adjust comparisons for differences in severity of patient conditions (IOM, 1994b; Roos et al., 1995). Even with improvements, data collected for one purpose (e.g., claims administration) may remain questionable for other purposes (e.g., outcomes research) if they lack reliable information about patient medical status, processes of care, and other variables. The OTA, for example, warned that "focusing on this research method as a relatively simple, inexpensive first-line tool for answering comparative questions [about the effectiveness of treatment alternatives] is unwarranted" (OTA, 1994, p. 74).

7

Evaluating the Effects of Telemedicine on Quality, Access, and Cost

Does telepyschiatry provide more timely access to appropriate behavioral health services than conventional arrangements for patients in a remote rural community? How does it affect patients' health and well-being compared to the alternatives? How do costs compare? Are patients and clinicians satisfied with the services? Would they want to use them in the future? Why or why not? These are the kinds of questions that clinicians, patients, managers, and policymakers want answered about telemedicine.

This chapter focuses on questions about the quality, accessibility, cost, and acceptability of telemedicine services. Additional questions will, however, be relevant for some organizations, some communities, and some evaluations. For example, because many telemedicine programs also serve educational and administrative purposes, evaluations may reasonably seek to assess results in these areas. The committee's evaluation framework likewise provides for strategic objectives such as strengthening an organization's competitive positive. As described in Chapter 5, the evaluation domains proposed by the federal Joint Working Group on Telemedicine included the "health system interface." Differing in form but not significantly in substance, the committee's framework treats this domain as a set of intermediate technical, clinical, and administrative factors that need to be tracked and understood as part of an evaluation of quality, access, cost, and acceptability outcomes.

Broader community effects may also be considered in an evaluation. Policymakers may, for example, be interested in the effects of telemedicine on the survival of rural health care providers and the implications of such effects for the overall economic health of rural areas, including their ability to attract or maintain business, educational, and other resources (OTA, 1991; Council on Competitiveness, 1994; GAO, 1996). For any specific evaluation, the selection of measures and criteria will depend on the telemedicine application, the alternatives to which it is compared, the target clinical problems and populations, the setting, and similar factors.

EVALUATION CRITERIA AND QUESTIONS

As defined in Chapter 1, an *evaluation criterion* is a measure, indicator, standard, or similar basis for describing outcomes or making judgments. Because clinical telemedicine varies so much, the committee broadly interpreted its charge to propose a set of evaluation criteria related to its evaluation framework. Applications differ in the medical problems addressed, the evidence base for decisionmaking, and the diagnostic, therapeutic, and other strategies employed. It would have been far beyond the resources for this project to develop operational measures or standards of care specific to the array of teleradiology, teledermatology, telepsychiatry, home health, emergency care, and other applications described in this report.

Rather, the committee started with the set of basic questions about quality, access, and cost that guide much health services research, particularly in the interrelated fields of clinical evaluation and technology assessment (IOM, 1993b, 1995a). Although patient satisfaction measures may be incorporated into assessments of quality of care, particularly in managed care plans (Cleary and McNeil, 1988; Gold and Wooldridge, 1995), more specific questions about patient and clinician satisfaction and other perceptions are presented separately in this chapter. Questions about health outcomes are largely subsumed in the discussion of quality but also enter into assessments of cost-effectiveness.

Table 7.1 lists the broad categories of questions proposed by the committee. The importance of comparing telemedicine to an alter-

TABLE 7.1 Categories of Evaluation Questions for Comparing
Telemedicine to Alternative Health Services

---

1. What were the effects of the application on the clinical process of care compared to the alternative(s)?
2. What were the effects of the application on patient status or health outcomes compared to the alternative(s)?
3. What were the effects of the application on access compared to the alternative(s)?
4. What were the costs of the application for patients, private or public payers, providers, and other affected parties compared to the alternative(s)?
5. How did patients, clinicians, and other relevant parties view the application, and were they satisfied with the application compared to the alternative(s)?

NOTE: Each question assumes that an anlysis of results will control for or take into account severity of illness, comorbidities, demographic characteristics, and other relevant factors.

native is highlighted in each question. The note for the table emphasizes that the research design and analytic strategy will need to take into account and control for such factors as the initial condition of patients. Thus, each question should be read with the phrase *"other things being equal"* as an implicit preface.

The next sections of this chapter provide definitions, discuss key concepts, and present additional questions focusing on different aspects of quality, access, cost, and patient and clinician attitudes. These sections should be read in the context of the overall framework presented in Chapter 6. That is, relevant patient and organizational characteristics should be identified and considered as they might affect results. The level of an evaluation—whether it reflects a patient, corporate, or societal perspective—should also be identified. The fit between the project objectives and results and the evaluation sponsor's purposes or strategic plan also needs to be factored into the plan for analysis and the interpretation of results. The human and policy issues identified in Chapters 3 and 4 likewise warrant attention so that evaluation planning casts a wide net for possible benefits and costs of an application.

Some telemedicine evaluations will focus less on individual patients than on populations, including but not limited to those enrolled in managed care plans. Analyses may consider outcomes for an entire patient population or may concentrate on outcomes for the least healthy or most vulnerable groups in a population (e.g., elderly individuals, migrant workers). For example, a telemedicine application might target a high-risk group to test whether surveillance and early intervention could reduce hospitalization and net costs.

QUALITY OF CARE

The ultimate purpose of any medical care is to maintain or improve health and well-being. Thus, how clinical applications of telemedicine affect the quality of care and its outcomes is a central evaluative question—as it is for any health service.

Definitions and Concepts

As defined in Chapter 1, quality of care is "the degree to which health care services for individuals and populations increase the likelihood of desired health outcomes and are consistent with current professional knowledge" (IOM, 1990c).[1] A few points about this definition are worth noting.

First, the definition covers both individuals and populations and both current and potential users of health care. This is consistent with an increasing focus in health services research and health policy on how different clinical interventions, programs, and resources can be deployed to the greatest social advantage. Second, because the evidence base about what works in health care is still modest, the definition acknowledges the relevance of professional knowledge, which includes experience and judgment as well as the results of biomedical and clinical research. Third, as is traditional in the literature on quality of care, the definition encompasses the link between the processes and the outcomes of care (Donabedian, 1966, 1982, 1985), although the emphasis in recent years has been on the latter. Many studies of health care quality also search for structural aspects of quality, for example, characteristics of a health system's personnel or organization that are associated with better health outcomes and that can be incorporated into accreditation or credentialing pro-

---

[1]The discussion in this section draws on the Institute of Medicine's work over the past decade on quality of care, effectiveness research, and related topics (in addition to IOM, 1990c, see IOM, 1985, 1990a, 1991, 1992a).

grams. Finally, the definition deliberately omits resource constraints on the grounds that judgments of what constitutes excellent, acceptable, or unacceptable quality should be independent of constraints on resources. This does not, however, imply that decisionmakers can or should ignore resources in making decisions about what level of quality is desired and affordable.

In recent years, traditional quality assessment and assurance concepts and strategies in health care have been powerfully reshaped by proponents of continuous quality improvement or total quality management models. These models stress internal responsibility for quality rather than external regulation. As noted in Chapter 6, they also posit planning, control, assessment, and improvement activities grounded in statistical and scientific precepts and driven by data.

Conventionally, three broad types of quality problems have been differentiated. They are *overuse of care* (e.g., unnecessary telemedicine consultations); *underuse of care* (e.g., failure to refer a patient for a necessary consultation); and *poor technical or interpersonal performance* (e.g., incorrect interpretation of pathology specimen or inattention to patient concerns). In principle, no one of these three problems is more important than any other. Depending, however, on the setting, the clinical condition, the predominant financing mechanism, and other circumstances, one area may warrant more attention than another in a particular telemedicine evaluation. For instance, as discussed in Chapter 4, policymakers have been concerned that payment for telemedicine in a fee-for-service context might lead to excessive consultations that might, in turn, lead to overuse of diagnostic or therapeutic services for which the benefit would not be worth the risk. In capitated environments, the worry has been that financial incentives might lead to underuse of appropriate face-to-face consultations or other services and to poorer performance in the interpersonal aspects of patient care, including good communication between clinician and patient.

For purposes of this discussion and consistent with past usage in IOM reports, *appropriate care* is defined as care for which "the expected health benefit [exceeds] the expected negative consequences by a sufficient margin" that the care is worth providing (Park et al., 1986, p. 6). At what point is the extra margin of expected benefit such that an intervention might be "worth" any additional risk, therefore making the intervention appropriate? Answering this question necessarily involves subjective—and sometimes controversial—judgments as well as objective clinical information. Such judgments may be arrived at through expert consensus processes or by reference to other interventions that have been accepted as standard practice.

The clinical effects of telemedicine applications can be measured and compared at several levels. One may, for example, look for effects on the process of care or for effects on the outcomes of care or both. In a discussion of the impact of diagnostic technologies, Fineberg and colleagues (1977) distinguished several process and outcome dimensions that might appropriately be assessed by evaluators. These dimensions include

- technical capacity—whether a technology is safe, accurate, and reliable (e.g., how do transmitted digital images compare to films?);
- diagnostic accuracy—whether a technology contributes to a correct diagnosis (e.g., was an initial dermatology diagnosis by a primary care clinician corrected after review by a dermatologist?);
- diagnostic impact—whether a technology provides diagnostic information that is useful in making a diagnosis (e.g., after the telemedicine consult, is a face-to-face consultation still necessary?);
- therapeutic impact—whether a technology influences patient management or therapy (e.g., do paramedics perform better when they have access to emergency cardiac telemetry?); and
- patient outcome—whether a technology improves patients' health and well-being (e.g., are postsurgical patients telemonitored in a nursing home more or less likely to develop wound infections than patients remaining in the hospital?).

The first four dimensions involve processes of care. The last involves outcomes. Both categories figure in the question set presented below.

In principle, several kinds of process and outcomes measures might be relevant for any specific telemedicine application. For example, in North Carolina, researchers studying an emergency medicine project involving rural emergency departments and four medical schools plan to collect process of care, utilization, and outcomes data on "patient flow, time to diagnosis, effectiveness of specialty consultation, types of cases, appropriateness of intervention at local levels, and patient stabilization" (Evaluation Plan of the North Carolina Emergency Consult Network, p. 2).

Questions about Quality of Care and Patient Outcomes

As explained above, the committee concluded that it would identify basic questions about quality of care to guide evaluators in devising questions and criteria specific to their telemedicine project, its objectives, and its context. Table 7.2 lists these questions. Some measures such as survival appear to have limited relevance for most telemedicine uses, although mortality measures might be considered in evaluating certain applications in emergency care and home monitoring.

Processes of Care

The first set of measures in Table 7.2 relate to processes of care. Process of care measures are useful in their own right as they help evaluators to understand how care is provided, how an intervention changes other aspects of the care process, and how processes of care might be improved to achieve better outcomes or greater efficiency (Donabedian, 1966, 1982; IOM, 1990a; Wilson and Cleary, 1995; Wilson and Kaplan, 1995).

It is important to note that the process measures discussed here do not cover a variety of important but often routine quality assurance procedures. For example, those involved with digital radiology and teleradiology have developed and are still improving quality assurance methods for testing, calibrating, and otherwise monitoring and maintaining equipment at central and remote sites (Forsberg, 1995).

Sometimes, process measures are employed as proxies for health outcomes when data on the latter are limited or unavailable. For example, an early retrospective evaluation of Army telemedicine in Somalia and other sites was able to determine whether the diagnosis or patient care plan changed after the telemedicine consultation, but evaluators lacked data to judge whether the change made a difference in patient outcomes (Walters, forthcoming). Difference in diagnosis may be the most common outcomes-related measure found in tele-medicine evaluations to date. Ideally, previous research should

TABLE 7.2 Evaluating Quality of Care and Health Outcomes

What were the effects of the telemedicine application on the clinical process of care compared to the alternative(s)?

Was the application associated with differences in the use of health services (e.g., office visits, emergency transfers, diagnostic tests, length of hospital stay)?

Was the application associated with differences in appropriateness of services (e.g., underuse of clearly beneficial care)?

Was the application associated with differences in the quality, amount, or type of information available to clinicians or patients?

Was the application associated with differences in patients' knowledge of their health status, their understanding of the care options, or their compliance with care regimens?

Was the application associated with differences in diagnostic accuracy or timeliness, patient management decisions, or technical performance?

Was the application associated with differences in the interpersonal aspects of care?

What were the effects of the telemedicine application on immediate, intermediate, or long-term health outcomes compared to the alternative(s)?

Was the application associated with differences in physical signs or symptoms?

Was the application associated with differences in morbidity or mortality?

Was the application associated with a difference in physical, mental, or social and role functioning?

Was the application associated with differences in health-related behaviors (e.g., substance abuse)?

Was the application associated with differences in patient satisfaction with their care or patient perceptions about the quality or acceptability of the care they received?

NOTE: Each question assumes that analysis of results will control for or take into account severity of illness, comorbidities, demographic characteristics, and other relevant factors.

have demonstrated a link between the proxy variable and the desired health outcome. Depending on the objective of an evaluation, the nature of the clinical problem and the intervention, and the resources and data available, the same variable (e.g., vaccination rates) may be treated as an outcome in some studies and as a process measure in others.

Characteristics of a specific telemedicine project may affect the interpretation of utilization and other process information. For example, given similar patient populations, one might expect an experienced primary care physician to refer fewer patients for specialty consultations than a nurse practitioner. One hypothesis for exploration is that the utility of telemedicine is greater when the (initial) difference between the skills and experience of consultant and the referring clinician is greater.

Outcomes of Care

The value of process measures notwithstanding, decisionmakers, clinicians, and patients have increasingly demanded information on outcomes and questioned the assumption that conformance to procedural standards equates to good health outcomes (Relman, 1988; IOM, 1990c; Lansky, 1993). As suggested in Table 7.2, measures of patient outcomes may focus on

- clinical status (physiological and cognitive);
- mental and emotional well-being;
- feelings of energy and vitality; or
- functional capacity (e.g., ability to perform various tasks related to personal life or employment).

Patient outcomes are generally considered to include not just desired endpoints of health care (e.g., reduced mortality, improved functioning) but also a broad range of immediate and intermediate results (e.g., reduced blood pressure, higher vaccination rates, fewer hospital readmissions for surgical complications) (Brenner et al., 1995). Because patient outcomes data are often difficult to obtain for longer-term outcomes and outcomes that occur outside the hospital, immediate or intermediate clinical results (e.g., physiological signs such as blood pressure or postoperative complications) are frequently used in place of longer-term results. The advantage of such measures is that they may be more directly and strongly linked to elements of a clinical intervention. Their great disadvantage is that their relationship to outcomes of greater relevance to patients (e.g., function) may be theoretical rather than documented through prior research.

The longer the interval that defines an episode of care or a long-term outcome and the more sources of care (and record systems) involved, the more difficult it is to obtain information. Eventually, the integrated, longitudinal computer-based patient record should overcome some of the difficulties in securing satisfactory shorter- and longer-term outcomes data.

A very large literature has accumulated on categories of health outcomes and the tools for measuring them (see, e.g., the quality primer in IOM, 1990c, Vol. II; Lohr, 1992; McDowell and Newall, 1993; CHPS, 1995; Fowler, 1995). Tools for assessing clinical performance and health outcomes have progressed considerably in recent years as methodologists and researchers have tested and improved the validity and reliability of measures and made them more relevant and usable in routine clinical practice. For example, health services researchers have developed shorter and more easily used instruments to measure health status. They also have devised both generic measures and more focused instruments for specific clinical conditions (e.g., diabetes) and settings (e.g., ambulatory care).

Each telemedicine evaluation will have to select quality and outcomes measures that fit the patients, settings, services, desired outcomes, and other characteristics of its project. In some cases, well-established instruments (e.g., for measuring depression or determining patients' assessment of their quality of life) may be available and appropriate for measuring patient outcomes. In other cases, evaluators will have to create measures and data collection instruments, with less confidence in their validity and reliability (see the last section of this chapter).

Adjustments for Patient Risk or Severity of Illness

Proper interpretation of patient outcomes data requires good information on patient characteristics, in particular, their health status. Comparisons of clinical interventions or programs should be adjusted statistically to account for differences in patient risk factors. These adjustments are also essential for proper interpretation of comparisons involving the costs of patient care alternatives.

Various schemes have been devised to measure and adjust for differences in the seriousness of patients' medical status (Thomas and Ashcraft, 1989, 1991; Iezzoni, 1992; Hopkins and Carroll, 1994). Some focus on care settings (e.g., intensive care units) whereas others are more general. Some are designed less for quality assessment purposes than for assuring that capitated, per case, or other payment mechanisms do not pay too much for healthier than average patients and too little for sicker patients. Debate continues on the strengths and limitations of different strategies, but the committee stresses the importance of attempting to identify and adjust for differences in patient status.

Other Quality of Care Issues

As noted elsewhere in this report, primary care physicians or nurse practitioners who participate with patients in telemedicine consultations may learn more about clinical problems that they once referred to specialists and, thereby, become more proficient at identifying and managing repeat problems on their own. Telemedicine may, in this respect, be analogous to the informal "curbside" consultation about a specific patient, a process that clinicians may value more highly than consulting a journal or undertaking formal continuing medical education.

The extent to which clinical applications of telemedicine have this kind of educational effect is not well documented. The committee believes this area warrants further study. Such study should consider not only changes in knowledge but also changes in practice and, preferably, in short- or long-term health outcomes. In addition, systems-oriented evaluations may be warranted to identify how telemedicine systems can support local quality improvement activities through (a) access to data resources, medical literature, and expert opinion, (b) focused educational interventions and mentoring initiatives; and (c) interorganizational collaborations.

Another question related to the impact of telemedicine use on users' knowledge or skills is whether clinicians become more skilled in telemedicine (e.g., relating more effectively to patients during interactive video consultations, reading transmitted images more accurately) as they use a particular application more often. Does some kind of learning curve exist for certain applications? If so, would studies find that a higher volume of use was associated with better outcomes beyond the learning period?[2] What might this imply for

---

[2]Interest in the link between volume and quality of care has arisen primarily in the context of selected surgical and other procedures. Evidence suggests that surgeons who routinely perform a large number of certain relatively complex procedures tend to have better outcomes than those performing such procedures only occasionally (Flood et al., 1984; Hughes et al., 1987; Luft et al., 1987; Hannan et al., 1989; Woods et al., 1992; Hannan et al., 1992). Some

programs with persistently low numbers of telemedicine consultations? Might some minimum number of cases be suggested as a floor? More generally, what kind of procedures, if any, are appropriate for training and then certifying proficiency in a particular telemedicine application?

How the volume-outcome hypothesis might apply for telemedicine is largely unexplored. One possibility is that quality of care would improve if the consultations involved both high-volume consultants and services those for which high volume was linked to better outcomes. Another possibility is that specialists who had received referrals that were subsequently handled through telemedicine consultation (with a different specialist) might lose the volume of cases needed to maintain their proficiency in diagnosing or treating certain problems. Even if local specialists were reasonably available, would more complex cases be diverted to distant telemedicine consultants? These unanswered questions have implications for both quality of care and access to care. The latter topic is discussed next.

EVALUATING ACCESS

From its beginnings, one of the major promises of telemedicine has been that it would improve access to health services for people living in rural or remote areas where medical professionals and facilities were scarce or altogether absent. This promise has been the rationale behind three decades' worth of demonstration projects targeted at rural areas. More recently, the potential for telemedicine to improve access for other groups—for example, the inner-city poor and the urban and suburban homebound—has attracted interest. An emerging issue is how a restructured health care system might employ telemedicine as part of increasingly aggressive strategies to manage patient access to services, especially hospital care and referrals to specialists.

Although the emphasis in telemedicine has been on geography or distance from health care providers as a barrier to timely care, other barriers to access also need to be considered in an evaluation frame-

---

health plans attempt to concentrate patients needing a complex procedure in a few "centers of excellence" that perform the procedure frequently, present evidence of good outcomes, and offer an attractive price.

work (IOM, 1993a,b) A more comprehensive list of barriers would include

• significant distance from primary, secondary, and tertiary medical services;
• poor transportation (e.g., lack of an automobile, limited or nonexistent bus service), even for relatively short distances;
• inadequate financial resources, particularly insurance coverage or directly subsidized services;
• family, educational, and cultural factors (e.g., illiteracy, distrust of technology);
• delivery system characteristics, including poor coordination of care, long waiting times for appointments, inadequate numbers or kinds of specialists, and bureaucratic obstacles to services; and
• gaps in our knowledge about how these factors interact to affect the use of services and what can be done to overcome or eliminate barriers to access.

Further, access involves more than an open door to personal health services provided by health professionals. Today, telecommunications and information technologies permit greater access to health information and thereby allow patients, potential patients, and families to learn more about health problems, care options, and prevention strategies. For those without computers or even telephones, however, access to these information resources is more a promise than a reality. Community clinics may be able to provide some with access to information resources, but funding for such services and for the clinics themselves is vulnerable to retrenchment in public services and budgets. Deficits in literacy and language skills may create further difficulties for disadvantaged populations. The gap in access may actually widen if information services improve only for the more affluent and educated.

The committee notes that the availability of telemedicine for clinical, educational, and other purposes may aid in the recruitment and retention of health professionals in underserved areas, although this has not yet been systematically evaluated. Telemedicine has the potential to tie rural practitioners more closely to experts and colleagues in more urban areas and, thus, to reduce isolation. To the extent that managed care networks reduce professional opportunities in urban and suburban communities and drive physicians and others to consider practice in underserved areas, clinical and educational uses of telemedicine could provide social and intellectual support that would ease such relocations.

Definitions and Concepts

Access was defined in Chapter 1 as the timely receipt of appropriate health care. More informally, access might be described as the availability of the right care at the right time without undue burden. The latter conceptualization maintains the notions of timeliness and appropriateness but adds two elements to the understanding of access: availability and burden.

One element, availability, incorporates the notion of services that stand ready for use *if and when needed*. Residents of an area may be considered to have access to available services (e.g., a nearby emergency department) even if most people never need or use them. The other element in the informal definition, undue burden, suggests that the difficulty of actually obtaining appropriate services should be considered in evaluating access. For example, if a telepsychiatry consultation saves a patient and others a risky trip over bad winter roads, then it has affected access. Similarly, if telemedicine helps ventilator-dependent patients avoid the burden of transport from the home to a physician's office, then access is affected. What constitutes an undue burden will clearly vary across individuals with differing incomes, insurance coverage, transportation resources, physical limitations, employment situations, and other characteristics. Whether a reduced burden for a patient is worth the cost involved is an important but separate question.

Both formal and informal conceptualizations of access imply that the evaluative focus ought to be on people's ability to get appropriate care rather than on their ability to get any service, whether appropriate or not. Although this point is easy to make, it is more difficult to translate into operational measures, in part because of disagreement about what constitutes appropriate care for specific problems and in part because of the difficulty of data collection or interpretation. As a result, resources (e.g., hospital beds or physicians per 1,000 population) are often used as indicators and may be acceptable for some evaluations. Nonetheless, the use of such measures may erroneously imply to some that more physical resources automatically equate to more health benefit.

One additional distinction may need to be considered. That is, does a telemedicine application affect access only when it directly involves the patient (e.g., as does an interactive video consultation for a psychiatric problem) or does it also affect access when mediated through a clinician (e.g., as in the typical teleradiology consultation)? If telemedicine allows a clinician quicker access to important information that would support a decision to treat locally rather than transfer or refer, then the patient could be said to have more timely access to appropriate care and, thus, better access to care.

Clearly, access as defined here involves multiple dimensions, some of which (e.g., appropriate care) overlap with quality and cost evaluations. Moreover, the committee recognizes that transforming concepts such as "timely," "appropriate," and "undue burden" into operational measures and evaluating results may involve considerable subjective judgment.

Questions about Access to Care

Table 7.3 lists the questions related to access proposed by the committee. Again, the choice, formulation, and interpretation of specific questions will depend on the type of application, the context in which it is employed, the research design, and the resources available for evaluation. Some questions may overlap with those used in evaluating other outcomes, such as patient satisfaction.

In principle, access may be measured at the individual, group, or the population level. Because access questions are often raised in the context of concerns about disadvantaged groups, the policy and evaluation focus is, in fact, often on populations or population subgroups. A 1993 IOM report on indicators of access to health care identified several population-based utilization and outcomes measures that could be employed to monitor national access objectives (often with a focus on identified problem groups such as rural or minority populations). For example, one proposed indicator of the lack of access to timely and appropriate treatment was avoidable hospitalization for chronic diseases. The suggested measures for this indicator included admission rates for selected ambulatory-care-sensitive conditions (e.g., asthma, diabetes) as determined from hospital discharge abstracts for groups defined by income (based on zip code

TABLE 7.3 Evaluating Access to Care

Did telemedicine affect the use of services or the level or appropriateness of care compared to the alternative(s)?
What was the utilization of telemedicine services before, during, and after the study period for target population and clinical problem(s)?
When offered the option of a telemedicine service, how often did patients
- accept or refuse an initial service or fail to keep an appointment
- accept or refuse a subsequent service or fail to keep an appointment?
What was the utilization of specified alternative services before, during, and after the study period for the target population and clinical problem(s)?
- consultants traveling to distant sites
- patients traveling to distant consultants
- consultation by mail or courier
- transfers to other facilities
- self-care
Was the telemedicine application associated with a difference in overall utilization (e.g., number of services or rate) or indicators of appropriateness of care for
- specialty care
- primary care
- transport services
- services associated with lack of timely care?

Did the application affect the timeliness of care or the burden of obtaining care compared to the alternative(s)?
Was there a difference in the
- timing of care
- appointment waiting times for referrals?
What were patient attitudes about the
- timeliness of care
- burden of obtaining care
- appropriateness of care?
What were the attitudes of attending and consulting physicians and other personnel about the
- timeliness of care
- burden of providing care
- appropriateness of care?

NOTE: Each question assumes that an analysis of results will control for or take into account severity of illness, comorbidities, demographic characteristics, and other relevant factors.

information).   Other access indicators included rates of vaccine-preventable childhood diseases and rates of immunizations.   For all such indicators and measures, the 1993 report discussed the nature and limits of available data sources.

Telemedicine remains at such an early stage of implementation and diffusion that the committee would not expect it to have had effects that would be evident from such population-based analyses. Furthermore, information on the use of telemedicine services is not routinely available in major national databases so that it would not now be possible to link the availability of telemedicine in different areas to differences in access measures.   The kinds of routine and specialized surveys and other data collection instruments used to obtain information for the databases described in the IOM report on access may, however, provide useful models for those devising measurement and data collection strategies for telemedicine projects employed by health systems that serve well-defined populations. Even so, relatively few clinics, health plans, or organizations have the combination of reasonably well-defined patient or enrollee populations, detailed clinical and administrative databases, and resources for special surveys that more sophisticated measures of access would require.

In reviewing telemedicine evaluation activities, the committee identified several access-related indicators that evaluators had used or hoped to obtain through existing or specially created data collection processes.   These indicators, which do not—in and of themselves—consider the appropriateness of services, include

- use of telemedicine services over time;
- changes in the number of traditional consultations;
- changes in waiting time for specialist appointments;
- changes in rates of missed appointments for consultations;
- patient willingness to participate in a telemedicine consultation; and
- patient or clinician attitudes about the timeliness of consultations and the burden of different consultation options.

Particularly with the increase in competition in the health care system, health care organizations have established a variety of performance indicators related to certain dimensions of access.   These include the wait time for different kinds of services (e.g., urgent versus nonurgent problems), time "on hold" for a telephone call, number of calls lost, and frequency of busy signals. What constitutes acceptable performance appears to vary depending on purchaser and patient expectations, regulations, resources, and other factors.

EVALUATING COSTS AND COST-EFFECTIVENESS OF TELEMEDICINE[3]

Although improved access to health care has been the motivating force behind many telemedicine applications, reduced health care costs or reduced rates of cost escalation have dominated many other health care initiatives. These include efforts to increase competition in health services, to change methods for paying clinicians and institutions, to make patients more conscious of costs, and to identify and discourage overuse of health services. In this environment, the costs and cost-effectiveness of telemedicine applications compared to conventional health services are understandably central concerns of decisionmakers.

Level and Perspective of the Analysis

As discussed generally in Chapter 6, it is essential to specify the level and perspective of an analysis and to include or exclude costs accordingly. Most relevant for many public policy decisions is the *societal* perspective, which encompasses the total costs of resources used to provide a service through telemedicine or alternative means. Nonetheless, it may also be appropriate for such analyses to identify how monetary costs and savings are distributed among particular parties. Entities such as insurers, providers, and patients bear variable portions of total costs and reap variable amounts of any cost savings.

Thus, an analysis based on a private insurer's perspective might incorporate costs only for health care benefits or services covered by the insurance plan and exclude any deductibles and copayments or uncovered medical and other expenses (e.g., transportation) borne

---

[3]This section is based in part on a paper drafted by committee members Jane Sisk and Jay Sanders.

by the insured and any bad debts absorbed by providers for patients who could not pay their share of costs. Hospitals and physician groups would generate a somewhat different set of included and excluded costs, as would patients. Moreover, in addition to costs for uncovered services and copayments or coinsurance, patients and other members of the population at risk experience health effects—positive and negative.

For health plans or providers paid on a capitation basis, the perspectives of payers and providers may be melded and reshaped as these parties assume financial responsibility for a comprehensive set of benefits for a defined population at risk. As discussed in Chapter 4, the financial incentives of capitation reward providers for delivering care in the most efficient manner. If telemedicine offers efficiencies compared to its alternatives, managed care plans and capitated systems are more likely to realize these benefits and to invest in telemedicine technologies. Further, to the extent that managed care and capitated delivery systems encompass a broader range of services and health professionals and to the extent that they maintain a stable enrollee population over time (which cannot be assumed), they may come closer than traditional insurers and providers to internalizing the total costs of alternative ways of managing medical conditions.

The perspective of analysis may be particularly important in the treatment of transportation costs. Health care organizations, integrated delivery systems, and managed care plans may or may not internalize the travel costs of physicians and other health professionals delivering care to people at a distance. Within traditional fee-for-service payment and private indemnity insurance, it has been unusual for plans to cover transportation of patients, except for ambulances or other special vehicles and for emergencies. However, some public programs, such as Medicaid, have covered more routine patient transportation, even under fee-for-service arrangements. For states, the prospect of reduced transportation costs has been a major attraction of prison telemedicine programs.

Definitions and Concepts

Costs are intended to measure the value of resource use associated with an intervention. The hallmark of economic evaluation is comparison of the costs and benefits of alternative ways of managing a condition. *Cost-effectiveness analysis*, the most common technique, compares costs and health effects of at least two alternatives. For example, a psychiatric consult or counseling session conducted through telemedicine could be compared to one conducted in person. Cost-effectiveness analysis expresses health effects in natural units, such as years of life gained or cases of cancer prevented.[4] By contrast, *cost-benefit analysis* expresses both costs and benefits (e.g., years of life gained) in monetary terms. The following discussion generally reflects basic principles of cost and cost-effectiveness analysis as identified in a number of sources (see, e.g., Weinstein and Stason, 1977; Warner and Luce, 1982; Drummond et al., 1987; Eisenberg, 1989; Sisk, 1990; Udvarhelyi et al., 1992; Kee, 1994; OTA, 1994).

It is not meaningful to question whether telemedicine per se is a good investment, because its worth—like that of any technology—depends on the circumstances of its use. The meaningful issue for evaluation is whether telemedicine is a good investment for a specific purpose, compared to an alternative(s). Ideally, an evaluation should specify the full range of actual alternatives, so that the results are relevant to the decisions that people face.

To calculate the total cost of telemedicine, one should, in principle, include the costs of all resources to all parties. Cost calculations should also factor in any savings or changes in productivity associated with the application. For example, the potential economic benefits of digital radiology networks include increases in the average number of images read per radiologist per week and reductions in the number of retaken or mislaid images, the times for image location and retrieval, and the physical space required for storage (Vanden and Strauss, 1995). Such benefits may be highly dependent on the technical characteristics and scope of an installation, for example, whether digital imaging is used on an institution-wide rather than supplemental or incremental basis or whether any major infrastructure costs are shared with other applications.

Capital costs for building, major remodeling, or large equipment expenses should be included if the project calls for telemedicine ca-

---

[4]Some analysts use the term *cost-utility analysis* when outcomes are expressed in units (e.g., quality-adjusted life years or QALYS) that are intended to apply commonly across different problems (OTA, 1994).

pacity to be established anew or for existing capacity to be significantly expanded. If a telemedicine project is operational, it may be appropriate to include only *variable* costs, that is, costs that vary with the level of output, such as the number of radiology consults or counseling sessions per month.

Cost analyses examine the differential, incremental, or *marginal* costs of one alternative compared to another. If the alternatives (e.g., telemedicine, mail, or personal travel for radiology consults) all equally use the same buildings and certain personnel, then the costs of those common resources will not affect comparative costs and need not be calculated for comparative analysis. The analysis should then focus on costs that differ among the alternatives, including personnel, supplies, and personal transportation and time for the radiologist or patient.

For a telemedicine application that requires an infrastructure with sizable fixed costs that cannot be legitimately shared or assigned in part to other users, the application of these principles implies a higher per unit cost. Similarly, during the start-up period of a program, spreading costs over a small number of cases will also result in high per unit costs. Such costs should decline as technological developments reduce infrastructure costs and make telemedicine more convenient for larger numbers of patients. For example, as health care organizations continue to computerize their medical records and as consumers acquire interactive devices for entertainment or personal communication (e.g., two-way cable services, computer access to the Internet), the costs of adding certain telemedicine services in institutions, offices, and homes will be reduced. (A related but distinct issue is that if parts of the telemedicine infrastructure are subject to rapid obsolescence and need replacing or upgrading, then costs may not decline as much.)

If the health effects or cost implications of telemedicine or its alternatives stretch over time, the future stream of health effects and costs should be discounted to their present value. *Discounting* reflects the idea that people place a higher value on events or benefits in the present than in the future and that funds invested in the present can reap interest over time. It is not an adjustment for inflation.

Though often used as proxies for the cost of services, "billed charges" are list prices that may contain substantial distortions among services, particularly given the discounted, per case, or other payment arrangements that now apply for a substantial portion of health services. Payments, which are based on actual financial transactions, are usually preferable to charges, although in markets characterized by deep discounts to some payers, they too may be a poor proxy for direct measures of costs. Capitated payments or payments for packages of services, such as diagnosis-related groups (DRGs), however, may not vary with changes in resource use and cost. Documenting the actual use and per unit cost of resources to provide a service is clearly the preferable approach, though much more difficult to do (see, e.g., Williams, 1996).

Conceptual Challenges

Cost analyses of telemedicine face certain conceptual challenges that typify new device-based technologies with sizable fixed costs and multiple potential uses. Cost analyses can address these issues and clarify their implications but cannot definitively resolve them.

One difficulty arises from the varied uses to which a telemedicine system may be put. Parts of the system might be used to support emergency medical services, radiology consults, interactive patient counseling sessions, and monitoring of patients in their homes. Although each application may have costs specific to its use, such as certain personnel and supplies, all the applications may share other costs related to certain equipment and perhaps certain personnel and supplies. In contrast to accounting conventions, which apply administrative rules to apportion such joint costs of production, economic principles call for allocating joint costs according to the demand that each service faces (OTA, 1980; Sisk et al., 1991).

Another challenge arises because telemedicine, like other innovations, may lead to expanded indications for use. For example, a telemedicine system may be established to permit more timely diagnosis and treatment of trauma patients in rural areas. Once available and accepted, however, primary care physicians may use telemedicine for less urgent cases that they once handled on their own. Even if per unit costs of telemedicine decline with the greater volume, total use and total expenditures may increase.

A third—and by now familiar—challenge is that technological change may render a static study of benefits, harms, and costs outdated, even before the analysis is completed. The diffusion and evolution of technologies, such as those used in telemedicine, is a dynamic process that calls for ongoing evaluation. As adoption and use proceed, telemedicine users are likely to gain greater experience and proficiency that, in turn, may be reflected in lower costs and better outcomes.

To better inform decisionmakers, the possibility of expanded indications or proficiency-related cost reductions may be modeled in a sensitivity analysis. As described in Chapter 6, if uncertainty surrounds the values of certain variables in the evaluation that are considered key, sensitivity analysis can vary the values over reasonable ranges. The findings will indicate how sensitive the results are to these uncertainties.

Question about Costs and Cost-Effectiveness

Table 7.4 summarizes the questions related to costs proposed by the committee. This summary does not distinguish between major categories of costs (e.g., fixed and marginal, capital and operating). Again, the selection of specific measures will depend on the type of application and the context in which it is employed.

Some of the questions in Table 7.4 highlight an important but difficult problem for evaluations of telemedicine and, indeed, evaluations of any new technology. That is, what was the effect of the technology on costs over an episode of acute or chronic illness? An evaluation that cannot link services and costs to such episodes may fail to identify care that prevents the need for later, more expensive care or, alternatively, causes a cascade of additional services. For example, home monitoring via telemedicine might encourage quicker identification and response to problems that might be costly to treat if not caught early. Alternatively, such monitoring might identify more borderline problems and generate more home or office visits (see, e.g., Weinberger et al., 1996). As noted elsewhere in this report, the longer the interval that should be tracked in an evaluation, the more difficult become the problems in collecting and properly attributing relevant data.

Decision Rules for Analyzing Cost-Effectiveness Results

For some patterns of cost-effectiveness results, the findings strongly suggest certain decisions. For example,

TABLE 7.4 Evaluating Health Care Costs and Cost-Effectiveness

What were the costs of the telemedicine application for participating health care providers or health plans compared to the alternative(s)?
Was an application associated with differences in attending clinicians' costs for personnel, equipment, supplies, administrative services, travel, or other items? Was an application associated with differences in revenues or productivity? What was the net effect?
Was an application associated with differences in consulting clinicians' or consulting organizations' costs for personnel, equipment, supplies, space, administrative services, travel, or other items? Was an application associated with differences in revenues or productivity? What was the net effect?
Was an application associated with differences in the cost per service, per episode of illness, or per member (health plan enrollee, capitated lives) per month?

What were the costs of the telemedicine application for patients and families compared to the alternative(s)?
Was the application associated with differences in direct medical costs for patients or families?
Was the application associated with differences for patients or families in other direct costs (e.g., travel, child care) or indirect costs (e.g., lost work days)?

What were the costs for society overall compared to the alternative(s)?
Was an application associated with differences in total health care costs, the cost per service, per episode of illness, or per capita?

How did the costs of the application relate to the benefits of the telemedicine application compared to the alternative(s)?

NOTE: Each question assumes that analysis of results will control for or take into account severity of illness, comorbidities, demographic characteristics, and other relevant factors.

• If an alternative is more costly and performs less well (e.g., produces fewer health benefits), it is undesirable.
• If an alternative is more costly and performs as well, it is undesirable.
• If an alternative is less costly and performs better, it should be used.

• If an alternative is less costly and performs as well, it should be used.

In other cases, cost-effectiveness results are more equivocal and judgments will be more subjective. For example,

• If an alternative is more costly and performs better, are the benefits gained worth the extra costs?
• If an alternative is less costly and performs less well, are the savings worth the health benefits foregone?

Some analysts have suggested ranges of costs that are considered reasonable, for example, a year of healthy life gained for less than $100,000 (Laupacis et al., 1992). Technology assessments often compare the cost for the option being evaluated to the cost for a well-established technology. Thus, the cost-effectiveness of population-based screening for prostate cancer might be compared to the cost-effectiveness of screening for cervical cancer. In general, cost-effectiveness analysis can guide, but not dictate, judgments about the reasonableness of costs for the health benefits obtained from different health technologies.

Decisionmakers must also consider budgetary limitations as well as cost-effectiveness. Indeed, it may well be that not all technologies considered to be cost-effective (e.g., that can gain a year of healthy life for less than $100,000) can be afforded, given the number of cases potentially involved and the total budgetary implications of different technologies.

PATIENT AND CLINICIAN PERCEPTIONS

The discussion of human factors in Chapter 3 stressed patient and clinician perceptions as they may affect the acceptance and adoption of telemedicine. This chapter has noted patient perceptions as a factor to be considered in evaluating quality, access, or cost-effectiveness. They are also important in their own right to the extent that successful telemedicine applications depend on patient and clinician acceptance.

Attempts to assess patient satisfaction or perceptions of quality derive in part from the consumer movement and quality improvement philosophies that have promoted patient autonomy, informed decisionmaking, and patient-centered care (see, e.g., President's Commission, 1983; Eddy, 1990; IOM, 1990c, 1992a; Kasper et al., 1992; and the sections on human factors and continuous quality improvement in Chapters 3 and 6, respectively). In recent years, increased competition in health care markets has also focused the attention of health plans, facilities, and clinicians on how patients or consumers view the quality, accessibility, or cost of the care they offer (Corrigan and Nielson, 1993; Gold and Wooldridge, 1995; Nelson et al., 1995). Employers and governments who purchase coverage for their employees or beneficiaries also have demanded such information. More generally, this is an era characterized by a steady stream of reports about reduced citizen trust in major social institutions and professions and increasing concern about the effect of managed care and selective contracting on physicians' allegiance to their patients. As a result, some effort may be warranted to assess patient trust in the clinicians and health care organizations involved in a telemedicine application.

Clinician perceptions are less often evaluated than patient perceptions, but efforts to improve the effectiveness or efficiency of care may depend on how satisfied those who provide care are with the conditions of practice (e.g., how convenient a telemedicine consultation is). In the committee's view, those evaluating telemedicine have been fairly sensitive to the clinician perspective. They have recognized that the special demands created by the complex and sometimes unfriendly technical infrastructure of telemedicine may frustrate clinicians, slow the provision of care, and create concerns about professional image. The discussion of human factors in Chapter 3 underscores the importance of considering clinician perspectives and needs.

In several telemedicine evaluations, patient satisfaction data appear to be the only patient-level data collected (ORHP, 1995). The committee considers this evaluative focus far too limiting, although it agrees that evaluators should consider patient—and clinician—views. The efforts by federal agencies to strengthen evaluations of federally funded telemedicine projects (as described in Chapter 5) reflects, in part, a recognition of the limitations of patient satisfaction data. Efforts to standardize questionnaires are also under way, as described in Chapter 5.

Methods and Focus

Attempts to assess patient or clinician perspectives usually involve written questionnaires. Questionnaires are attractive tools because they are relatively inexpensive and convenient to administer and analyze, especially if they can be computer scored. They are also relatively flexible and can be administered on-site, by mail, or by telephone, although the validity and reliability of different forms of administration needs to be considered on a case-by-case basis. Some questionnaires focus on discrete encounters (e.g., an office visit) whereas others focus on institutions or organizations (e.g., hospitals or health plans). For the immediate future, telemedicine evaluations will most likely focus on encounters.

The validity and reliability of various instruments for measuring patient satisfaction have been assessed, but more work remains to be done in general and with respect to specific populations, interventions, settings, and outcomes (Ware et al., 1988; Webster, 1989; Hall et al., 1990; IOM, 1990a; Rubin, 1990; Peterson and Wilson, 1992; Carey and Seibert, 1993; Rubin et al., 1993; Bayley et al., 1995; Gold and Wooldridge, 1995; Stump et al., 1995; Etter et al., 1996). Those who use surveys also have to be sensitive to the methodological problems frequently encountered in many kinds of survey research (e.g., nonresponse rates, accuracy of patient recall, positive response bias).

Telemedicine applications potentially offer an unusual opportunity to explore patient satisfaction data in more depth. Because telemedicine encounters may involve video records, it may be possible to match individual encounters with questionnaires and to assess the encounters qualitatively in light of the survey responses. In addition to providing feedback to clinicians and program administrators, evaluators could explore how such qualitative assessments could provide additional guidance about improving practices that appear associated with negative responses. Video taping and critiquing has become relatively common as a teaching tool for medical students. As is true for feedback strategies in general, evaluators would need to provide for appropriate patient consent and be prepared for clinician reaction to negative evaluations.

Questions about Patient and Clinician Perceptions

Tables 7.5 and 7.6 present general questions that may be asked about patient or clinician perceptions. The questions concerning patient satisfaction with telemedicine reflect the approach taken in the applicable Medical Outcomes Study (MOS) visit-specific questions. This approach has been extensively tested (Rubin et al., 1993; Bayley et al., 1995). Although the selection of specific questions will depend on the purposes of a particular evaluation, the design and administration of questionnaires should follow general principles of questionnaire construction (Rossi et al., 1983; Lessler, 1995).

Depending on the objectives of an evaluation, relatively general questions may be adequate. If, however, the objective is to pinpoint problems, then questions may need to be not only more specific but also more quantitative. For example, rather than ask generally about whether clinicians found the application convenient, questions might be asked about how much time the consultation took or about whether the hardware or software was difficult to manipulate and

TABLE 7.5 Evaluating Patient Perceptions

Were patients satisfied with the telemedicine service compared to the alternative(s)?

How did patients rate their physical and psychological comfort with the application?

How did patients rate the convenience of the encounter, its duration, its timeliness, and its cost?

How did patients (and family members) rate the skills and personal manner of the consultant and the attending personnel (e.g., primary care physician, nurse practitioner)?

Was the lack of direct physical contact with the distant clinician acceptable?

How did patients rate the explanations provided to them of what their problem was and what was being recommended?

Did patients have concerns about whether the privacy of personal medical information was protected?

Would patients be willing to use the telemedicine service again?

Overall, how satisfied were patients with the telemedicine services they received?

NOTE: Each question assumes that analysis of results will control for or take into account prior patient experiences with the health care system, severity of illness, comorbidities, demographic characteristics, and other relevant factors.

TABLE 7.6 Evaluating Clinician Perceptions

Were attending/consulting clinicians satisfied with the telemedicine
application compared to the alternative(s)?
How did attending/consulting clinicians rate their comfort with telemedicine
   equipment and procedures?
How did attending/consulting clinicians rate the convenience of telemedicine
   in terms of scheduling, physical arrangements, and location?
How did attending/consulting clinicians rate the timeliness of consultation
   results?
How did attending/consulting clinicians rate the technical quality of the
   service?
How did attending/consulting clinicians rate the quality of communications
   with patients?
Were attending/consulting clinicians concerned about maintaining the
   confidentiality of personal medical information and protecting patients'
   privacy?
Did attending/consulting clinicians believe the application made a positive
   contribution to patient care?
Would the clinicians be willing to use the telemedicine services again?
Overall, how satisfied were the attending/consulting clinicians with the
   telemedicine service?

NOTE: Each question assumes that analysis of results will control for or take into
account severity of illness, comorbidities, demographic characteristics, and other
relevant factors.

how much time was lost to such problems. In addition, in depth
interviews may be useful to develop a fuller understanding of how
people perceive the advantages and disadvantages of telemedicine.

   The consistency and stability of patient perceptions may warrant
particular attention. For example, one unpublished study of telecardiology patients found that patients did not find the experience
unpleasant (93 percent), an invasion of privacy (95 percent), or unacceptable for lack of physical contact (88 percent). Nonetheless,
only 67 percent said they would use the system for emergency or first
visits and only 51 percent wanted to use it for follow-up visits
(Mattioli, 1996). In an unpublished follow-up survey a year later
(which had a 54 percent response rate), a third of the respondents
said they would use the system only in an emergency and a third
would go elsewhere if it were their only option.

DESIRABLE ATTRIBUTES OF EVALUATION CRITERIA

Drawing on the work of several groups considering practical but systematic means of improving clinical practice and health care delivery (IOM, 1990c, 1992a,b; Medical Outcomes Trust, 1995; CPRI, 1996), the study committee identified several desirable characteristics or attributes of evaluation criteria (Table 7.7). These attributes are generic, that is, in principle, they should apply to quality, access, and cost criteria alike and to qualitative as well as quantitative measures. They are also *ideal* attributes; actual criteria will almost certainly fall short on at least some aspects.

For several of the attributes (including reliability and validity) and certain kinds of clinical measures, a *controlled vocabulary* (i.e., a precise, common clinical terminology) is important. The need for a controlled vocabulary arises from a common difficulty in clinical research, clinical practice guidelines, and medical informatics: the lack of unambiguous, uniform descriptors of patient problems (see IOM, 1990c, 1992a; Gibson and Middleton, 1994; Ozbolt et al., 1994). For example, terms like "moderate bleeding" or "persistent

TABLE 7.7 Desirable Attributes of Evaluation Criteria

Reliability/Reproducibility An evaluation instrument or criterion is reliable if repeated use under identical circumstances by the same or different users produces the same results.

Validity An evaluation instrument or criterion is valid if it measures the properties, qualities, or characteristics it is intended to measure.

Responsiveness An evaluation instrument or criterion is responsive if it can detect important differences in outcomes across evaluation groups or time periods.

Interpretability An evaluation instrument or criterion is interpretable if users find the results of its application understandable.

Feasibility An evaluation instrument or criterion is feasible if users can accomplish the required activities, collect the necessary information, and analyze the resulting data within available evaluation resources and without imposing excessive burdens on those whose cooperation is required for the evaluation.

Flexibility An evaluation instrument or criterion is flexible if it is adaptable to a variety of evaluation problems or circumstances.

Documentation An evaluation instrument or criterion is documented if the protocols for applying and interpreting it are specified and if evidence of its successful use is summarized or cited.

bleeding" may be interpreted differently in practice by different observers. Bleeding defined in terms of volume loss or hematocrit
drops is more precise. Even if definitions are unambiguous, a problem remains if they are not uniformly used. In this context, a
controlled vocabulary is one specified by those responsible for an
information system and one that precludes users from adding unauthorized terms.

Developing a controlled vocabulary and implementing it are long-
term challenges. Several schemes have been developed to increase
uniformity in the coding of patient history and physical results, medical diagnoses, or procedures. They go under a variety of abbreviations and acronyms (e.g., ICD-9-CM, CPT-4, SNOMEDIII) and are
described in detail elsewhere (e.g., PPRC, 1988; IOM, 1991; AMA,
1993; CAP, 1993; Gibson and Middleton, 1994). To build on these
efforts, the National Library of Medicine has developed a Uniform
Medical Language System (UMLS) Metathesaurus to map terms used
by such schemes.

CONCLUSION

This chapter has reviewed issues in measuring and evaluating
critical outcomes for telemedicine and proposed general evaluation
questions in four key areas: quality, access, cost, and patient and
clinician perceptions and satisfaction. Depending on the application
and clinical problem, the setting and patient population, the objectives of the program, and other factors, evaluations will differ in the
outcomes of greatest interest and relevance. As stressed in Chapter
6, the earlier and more precisely evaluation objectives and questions
are identified, the more likely it is that the program to be evaluated
can be designed and implemented in ways that will help provide
useful and credible answers.

Although the questions about quality, access, cost, and patient
and clinician perceptions are presented sequentially above, their in-
terrelationships also warrant attention. For example, the timeliness
of care—an element of access as defined here—may have important
consequences for quality through earlier detection and better management of clinical problems. Similarly, economic analyses of telemedicine do not simply examine costs but attempt to relate the costs
of an application to its benefits and to suggest bases for judging
whether the benefits are worth the costs in comparison to other

alternatives. Judgments are typically based on a balancing of objectives that is contingent on a given evaluation's mix of effects on quality, access, and cost. For evaluations that are beyond the "test of concept" or formative phase, a central question will often be: What do the quality, access, cost, and other results suggest about whether and how the telemedicine program can be sustained beyond the evaluation stage?

8

Findings and Recommendations

For some applications of telemedicine, more rigorous evaluations will support claims about their value and will encourage their more widespread use. For other applications, better evaluation may discourage adoption, at least until technologies and infrastructures improve or other circumstances change. That is to be expected. The purpose of evaluation—and the purpose of this report—is not to endorse telemedicine but to endorse the development and use of good information for decisionmaking.

The committee recognized that telemedicine applications—like other health services and technologies—will diffuse in some measure despite limited systematic assessment of their benefits and costs. This diffusion may also be marked by too much attention to the more glamorous but not necessarily more cost-effective technologies, although strong incentives to control costs may be weakening tendencies in this direction. Conversely, telemedicine applications may also languish for lack of good evidence documenting their relative value compared to alternative services or for lack of evaluation research identifying the obstacles standing in the way of useful and sustainable programs.

This final chapter builds on the preceding seven chapters. It begins by summarizing the technical and human factors and the policy context that may affect decisions about telemedicine. It next reviews challenges in evaluating telemedicine. The chapter then presents the evaluation principles set forth by the committee and a summary of the committee's evaluation framework and related recommendations and conclusions.

THE TECHNICAL, HUMAN, AND POLICY CONTEXT FOR TELEMEDICINE EVALUATIONS

Telecommunications and information technologies are evolving to provide and support medical care at a distance. Some of these technologies involve incremental improvements in the way familiar tools, such as the telephone, are used; others, such as telesurgery, involve devices and procedures that are still experimental.

The committee found general consensus about technical, behavioral, and policy factors that contribute to the modest implementation and documented success to date of the more technologically advanced forms of telemedicine. On the technical side, those responsible for deploying, sustaining, and managing information and telecommunications systems and programs face an often confusing array of constantly changing hardware and software options, many of which are not tailored to health care users. Assessing the utility of advanced technologies can be difficult, particularly given the frequent need to consider options in combination and not just individually. New systems generally have to be patched together with existing or legacy systems that cannot be immediately replaced. Although many groups are working to develop hardware and software standards, it remains frustrating and difficult to put together systems in which the components operate predictably and smoothly together and function in different settings without extensive adaptation.

The limited adoption of telemedicine also appears to stem from a variety of human factors. Research on factors affecting the acceptance of telemedicine is sparse, but the committee heard considerable consensus about practical, socioeconomic, and system constraints related to

- meager evidence for clinicians that an application will benefit them in their day-to-day practice;
- inadequate assessment of practitioner and community needs by those promoting telemedicine;
- practical difficulties in incorporating telemedicine into daily

Zaremba, L.A., and Anderson, M.P. Everything You Need to Know about FDA Regulation of PACS Equipment. Presentation at the Society for Computer Applications in Radiology meeting. Denver, June 1996.

Zaremba, L.A., and Phillips, R.A. Image Compression: Regulatory Issues and Policies. Presentation at the American Association of Physicists in Medicine Annual Meeting, Washington, D.C., 1993.

Zelen, M. Large Sample Trials: The Open Protocol System. In *Clinical Trials and Statistics: Proceedings of a Symposium.* Board on Mathematical Sciences, Commission on Physical Sciences, Mathematics, and Applications, National Research Council. Washington, D.C.: National Academy Press, 1993.

Zundel, K.M. Telemedicine: History, Applications, and Impact on Librarianship. *Bulletin of the Medical Library Association* 84(1):71–79, 1996.

Appendixes

A

Examples of Federal Telemedicine Grants

The following agencies and sponsored projects are included as a representative (but by no means comprehensive) listing of telemedicine activities.

OFFICE OF RURAL HEALTH POLICY (ORHP), DEPARTMENT OF HEALTH AND HUMAN SERVICES

The ORHP maintains 19 three-year telemedicine grants which totaled $6.9 million in FY 1994 and $7.6 million in FY 1995. The 12 projects receiving the largest awards are listed below.

MDTV, West Virginia University, Robert C. Byrd Health Sciences Center, Morgantown, West Virginia

Amount of award: $800,000 (1994), $800,000 (1995), and $800,000 (1996 request).

MDTV (Mountain Doctor Television) is adding several new sites in its fourth year of funding from ORHP. In addition to its two hub sites at Morgantown and Charleston and six rural spoke sites in New Martinsville, Gassaway, Buckannon, Elkins, Petersburg, and Madison, the West Virginia School of Osteopathic Medicine, Cabell

Huntington Hospital, a psychiatric facility, and two rural community health centers will join the network. In total, the network will have 15 sites throughout West Virginia. MDTV uses fully interactive audio and video and offers full consultative services. MDTV is also participating in a pilot project for the Health Care Financing Administration to test Medicare payment methodologies for telemedicine.

University of North Carolina at Chapel Hill, Department of
    Medicine, Program on Aging, Chapel Hill, North Carolina

Amount of award: $464,160 (1994), $409,431 (1995), and $437,321 (1996 request).

This project utilizes the North Carolina Information Highway (NCIH) to connect the University of North Carolina at Chapel Hill with three rural sites: Roanoke Amaranth Community Health Group, Our Community Hospital, and Halifax Memorial Hospital. Building on a five-year clinical program of interdisciplinary geriatric assessment, the fiber optic network will support interactive video consultations among the four sites.

Rapid City Regional Hospital, Rapid City, South Dakota

Amount of award: $460,680 (1994), $500,000 (1995), and $500,000 (1996 request).

This project supports three telemedicine networks in the state of South Dakota. The Rapid City Network became operational in February 1995 and is demonstrating store-and-forward technology for teleradiology and telecardiology with hospitals in Custer and Philip. The Sioux Valley Network has been operational since July 1994, demonstrating store-and-forward (for teleradiology) as well as interactive technologies. The McKennan Network began operations on January 1996. An evaluation of the project is being conducted by the South Dakota Department of Health.

Eastern Montana Telemedicine Network, Deaconess-Billings Clinic
    Health Systems, Billings, Montana

Amount of award: $334,000 (1994), $480,997 (1995), and $500,000 (1996 request).

The Eastern Montana Telemedicine Network uses two-way interactive video conferencing to deliver specialty care to ten geographically isolated communities in rural eastern Montana. The project has been partially funded with a grant from the Rural Utilities Service. Funding from the ORHP Rural Telemedicine Grant Program has been used to expand the project from four isolated rural communities to seven and to add another hub site at the Behavioral Health Clinic in Billings. Several of the rural counties served are Health Professional Shortage areas.

The Mid-Nebraska Telemedicine Network, Good Samaritan
    Hospital, Kearney, Nebraska

Amount of award: $479,060 (1994), $475,100 (1995), and $480,100 (1996 request).

The Mid-Nebraska Telemedicine Network is a consortium of five rural hospitals and Good Samaritan Health Systems (a regional referral center that includes Good Samaritan Hospital, an acute care facility, and Richard Young Hospital, a psychiatric and chemical dependency hospital). The system provides video conferencing and store-and-forward capabilities. During the first two months of operation, 31 patients were served, saving an average of 133 miles of driving under winter conditions.

Mary Imogene Bassett Hospital, New York

Amount of award: $259,415 (1994), $366,565 (1995), and $379,005 (1996 request).

Mary Imogene Bassett Hospital is developing a telemedicine system with two rural hospitals and fourteen rural outreach centers. Funds from the Rural Telemedicine Grant program will be used primarily for operating and evaluating the project that was initiated with a grant from the Rural Electrification Administration (now the Rural Utilities Service), U.S. Department of Agriculture.

REACH-TV, East Carolina University School of Medicine,
    Greenville, North Carolina

Amount of award: $438,970 (1994), $499,888 (1995), and $368,038 (1996 request).

REACH-TV (Rural Eastern Carolina Health Network) builds upon a network developed by the East Carolina University (ECU) Center for Health Sciences Communication and the Eastern Area Health Education Center. Funding from ORHP was used to support specialty consultations from ECU School of Medicine to Chowan Hospital in Edenton and Goshen Medical Center in Faison. The network will also be used by an interdisciplinary training program for preceptoring, conferencing, and consultations at Faison. Other aspects of this project include an ethnographic study of provider acceptance of telemedicine for psychiatric care, a school-based telehealth project in Plymouth, and a collaborative research project with Emory University in Georgia, evaluating the use of still-image telemedicine technologies. REACH-TV will also participate in a pilot project with HCFA to test Medicare payment methodologies for telemedicine.

High Plains Rural Health Network, Fort Morgan, Colorado

Amount of award: $499,056 (1994), $499,671 (1995), and $499,402 (1996 request).

The High Plains Rural Health Network provides interactive video conferencing to deliver specialty health care and continuing medical education to several medically underserved areas in Colorado, Nebraska, and Kansas. The network has three hub sites—Denver, Sterling, and Fort Collins—serving five rural spoke sites. Additional sites are becoming connected to the network as part of a recently awarded grant from the Rural Utilities Service. Over a half-dozen sites in Colorado will later be linked to the network through additional funding from a state grant.

Kentucky Telecare, University of Kentucky Medical Center,
    Lexington, Kentucky

Amount of award: $415,320 (1994), $482,988 (1995), and $477,243 (1996 request).

Kentucky Telecare is a partnership established to link rural primary care clinics, regional medical centers, and the University of Kentucky Medical Center. A video network currently operating in three rural communities provides clinical, educational, and administrative services. Over the next year, this system will extend to cover the entire Appalachian region and beyond, as seven more sites are added. Eleven primary care clinics will be equipped to transmit still images over telephone lines to the regional hubs.

University of Minnesota Telemedicine Project, Minneapolis, Minnesota

Amount of award: $294,052 (1994), $406,490 (1995), and $394,240 (1996 request).

The University of Minnesota Hospital and Clinic is connected to three rural sites in Wadena, Fergus Falls, and Staples. The network, operational since March 1995, has provided more than 100 interactive specialty consultations.

Missouri Telemedicine Network, University of Missouri-Columbia, Missouri

Amount of award: $411,124 (1994), $457,177 (1995), and $337,662 (1996 request).

This project uses two-way interactive television to link the University of Missouri Health Sciences Center with four rural hospitals and four primary care clinics. The Rural Telemedicine Grant funding served as a catalyst for obtaining additional private funding that supports expansion of the network to six additional rural hospitals, the Ellis Fischel Cancer Center, and the Kirksville College of Orthopaedic Medicine. All 17 sites in the network were scheduled to be operational by the end of summer 1996.

WAMI Rural Telemedicine Network, University of Washington School of Medicine, Department of Family Medicine, Seattle, Washington

Amount of award: $499,993 (1994), $499,993 (1995), and $499,993 (1996 request).

Four rural sites in four states—Washington, Alaska, Montana, and Idaho—are connected to the University of Washington School of Medicine in Seattle. The desktop video conferencing technology allows rural providers and patients to talk directly with consultants while electronically exchanging information and images such as charts or x-ray and MRI films.

NATIONAL LIBRARY OF MEDICINE (NLM), DEPARTMENT OF HEALTH AND HUMAN SERVICES

In 1995, the National Library of Medicine had contracts totaling $26 million for projects designed to help physicians practice better medicine by utilizing advanced computing and networking capabilities. As described in the *HPCC News*, a National Library of Medicine newsletter for the High Performance Computing and Communications program, the projects most directly involving telemedicine applications include the following.

Testbed Networks

Toward a National Collaboratory of Healthcare Informatics

This project is a collaboration involving three medical informatics research groups (Trustees of Columbia University, Brigham & Women's Hospital, and Board of Trustees of the Leland Stanford Junior University) to build Internet-accessible shared systems. The system will support computerized patient records, clinical research protocols, medical vocabulary servers, teleconferencing, and health professions education.

A Pilot Indianapolis-wide Megabit Network for Patient Care and Research

This project will tie together a major teaching hospital with community clinics and pharmacies, providing access to a computerized patient record system, computerized prescriptions, and on-line medical knowledge sources. The evaluation component will assess the cost and patient outcomes changes that result from the use of shared medical information.

A Chicago Metropolitan Medical Network

Northwestern Memorial Hospital is developing a testbed urban network that provides real-time access to patient clinical information and real-time consultation between linked sites and hospital-based specialists. The objectives of the project are to create information linkages between a hospital, physician offices and clinics, and a university medical school and library through the design and implementation of a technologically innovative and cost-effective communications network.

A High Performance Testbed Network for Telemanagement of Neuro-Imaging

A high-performance wide-area network will be used to transmit neuroradiology images for consultation, patient monitoring, and shared clinical management. This project will examine clinical outcomes that result from use of digital networks to transmit computed tomography and MRI of the brain and spinal cord.

Iowa Testbed Network

This project will use the newly developed, statewide digital network for creation of a Telecommunications Health Education Resource Center, for the linking of three hospital sites, for improved information services for rural health care providers, and for several telemedicine prototype systems.

Virtual Reality for Medicine

Organ Modeling in Support of Virtual Surgery Simulation

This project will create and evaluate advanced computer simulations of human anatomic structure which support surgical planning and health professions education.

Collaborative Technology for Real-time Treatment of Patients

A Comprehensive Teledermatology Program

This program of the Oregon Health Sciences University will involve the remote diagnosis of skin lesions via teleconsultation to primary care clinics in underserved rural areas of Oregon.

Implementation of a Teleradiology System to Enhance Consultative Services Between Primary and Secondary Care Hospitals and a Tertiary Care Facility

This project will link six outlying hospitals in western Pennsylvania with the University of Pittsburgh Medical Center for teleradiology to improve neurosurgery, neurology, trauma, and critical care. Impact of the system on patient outcomes will be studied.

Collaboration Technology for Real-time Treatment of Patients in West Virginia

A consortium of nine institutions led by the Concurrent Engineering Research Center of University of West Virginia will build and evaluate a regional telemedicine system for rural areas of the state.

Linking Images to a Clinical Information System

This project at the University of Pittsburgh will develop an "Image Engine" system for storing, retrieving, and sharing a wide range of clinically important images, integrating those images and dynamically linking them to data in the electronic record.

HEALTH CARE FINANCING ADMINISTRATION, DEPARTMENT OF HEALTH AND HUMAN SERVICES

Iowa Health System Telemedicine Demonstration

A grant was awarded in September 1993 for the "Evaluation of Clinical and Educational Services to Rural Hospitals via Fiber Optic Cable."

University of Michigan School of Public Health, Medical College of Georgia, and MDTV of West Virginia

This three-year project (sponsored at $1,265,651) consists of developing, testing, and implementing a detailed methodology for evaluating telemedicine. The Medical College of Georgia Telemedicine Center and MDTV at the University of West Virginia Health Sciences Center will provide study sites. A panel of experts will be appointed to develop a detailed methodology for telemedicine evaluation.

MDTV, West Virginia University, Robert C. Byrd Health Sciences Center, Morgantown, West Virginia

See description under ORHP. MDTV will be participating in a pilot project to test Medicare payment methodologies for telemedicine.

REACH-TV, East Carolina University School of Medicine, Greenville, North Carolina

See description under ORHP. Funding from the Health Care Financing Administration was used to connect ECU with two other rural sites. REACH-TV will also participate in a pilot project with HCFA to test Medicare payment methods for telemedicine.

NATIONAL TELECOMMUNICATIONS AND INFORMATION ADMINISTRATION, DEPARTMENT OF COMMERCE

City-County Health Department of Oklahoma County, Oklahoma

Amount of award: $128,970 (1994).

This project developed a plan to improve the department's surveillance and data systems. The objectives for an improved system include the ability for users to interconnect between different network systems, the establishment of new network capabilities and interconnections, and the establishment of a common database of demographic and geographic information that allows for surveillance of health risk factors, epidemiological studies, and promotion of community health.

Columbia University Health Sciences Division, New York

Amount of award: $733,424 (1994).

Columbia-Presbyterian Medical Center, the New York City Department of Health, and the Visiting Nurse Services of NYC collaborated to develop and demonstrate an information infrastructure to provide coordinated care to tuberculosis patients in the home, doctor's office, and hospital. The project used automated decision support systems, networks, interactive wireless hand-held computers, and natural language processing technology to coordinate the many providers of care for TB patients, ensure that the appropriate protocols were followed, develop an infrastructure that could be used in the treatment of other diseases, and document how electronic medical records can meet high standards of privacy and confidentiality.

Commonwealth of Pennsylvania

Amount of award: $379,302 (1994).

The Commonwealth of Pennsylvania will develop the Keystone State Desktop Medical Conferencing Network which will link physicians in rural/remote areas with resources in urban areas, including consulting physicians and medical libraries and databases. Three tertiary care facilities, a rural hub site, and ten rural physicians are participating.

Saint Louis University School of Public Health, Missouri

Amount of award: $136,966 (1994).

The Saint Louis Integrated Immunization Information System will provide all public health providers of immunization to children under age two in St. Louis with on-line real-time access to immunization information in hopes of raising the immunization rate.

B

Glossary* and Abbreviations

GLOSSARY

Advanced Research Projects Agency (ARPA). The DOD agency that created the computer network that evolved into the Internet.

Amplifier. Electronic devices used to boost the strength of a signal as it passes along a communications channel.

Analog signal. A continuous electrical signal in the form of waves that vary as the source of the information varies (e.g., as the contrast in an image varies from light to dark).

Architecture. The selection, design, and interconnection of the physical components of a computer system.

Asynchronous communication. Two-way communication in which there can be a time delay between when a message is sent and when it is received.

Asynchronous transfer mode (ATM). A type of switching that is expected to bridge the gap between packet and circuit switching. ATM uses packets called cells that are designed to switch cells so fast that there is no perceptible delay.

---

* Sources for these definitions, in addition to members of the committee, include ORHP, 1993; Greberman et al., 1994; OTA 1995; and the Telemedicine Glossary developed by the State University of New York Health Science Center at Syracuse (http://www.hscsyr.edu/wwwserve/telemedicine/glossary.html)

Audio-teleconferencing. Two-way electronic voice communication between two or more people at separate locations.

Authentication. The use of passwords, keys, and other automated identifiers to verify the identity of the person sending or receiving information.

Automated data collection. Direct transfer of physiological data from monitoring instruments to either a bedside display system or a computer-based patient record.

Backbone. A high-capacity communications channel that carries data accumulated from smaller branches of the computer or telecommunications network.

Bandwidth. A measure of the information carrying capacity of a communications channel; a practical limit to the size, cost, and capability of a telemedicine service.

Baud. A unit of digital transmission signaling speed of information transmission; the highest number of single information elements (bits) transferred between two devices (such as modems or fax machines) in one second.

Bell Operating Companies (BOCs). Grouped under the seven Regional BOCs (see RBOC).

Bit. Binary digit, the smallest possible unit of information making up a character or a word in digital code processed by computers.

Bps. The number of binary digits transmitted per second in a data communication system.

Broadband. Communications (e.g., broadcast television, microwave, and satellite) capable of carrying a wide range of frequencies; refers to transmission of signals in a frequency-modulated fashion, over a segment of the total bandwidth available, thereby permitting simultaneous transmission of several messages.

Byte. A set of eight bits.

Cable television (CATV). A transmission system that distributes broadcast television signals and other services by means of a coaxial cable.

Central processing unit (CPU). A unit of a computer that includes circuits controlling the interpretation and execution of instructions.

Channel. A radio frequency assignment made according to the frequency band being used and the geographic location of the sending/receiving sites.

Circuit Switched Network. A network that temporarily connects two or more channels between two or more points to provide the user with exclusive use of an open channel to exchange information, also called line switching and dial-up service.

Clinical information system. Hospital-based information system designed to collect and organize data related to the care given to a patient, rather than administrative data.

Coaxial cable. Transmission wire(s) covered by an insulating layer, a shielding layer, and an outer jacket; used for data, voice, and video transmissions; can transmit either broadband (several signals) or baseband (one signal).

Codec. A "code/decode" electrical device that converts an analog electrical signal into a digital form for transmission purposes and then converts it back at the other end.

Common carrier. A telecommunications company regulated by government agencies that offers communications relay services to the general public via shared circuits, charging published and nondiscriminatory rates.

Communication multiplexer. A device that allows data from multiple, lower speed communication lines to share a single higher speed communication path.

Compatibility. The ability for computer programs and computer readable data to be transferred from one hardware system to another without losses, changes, or extra programming.

Compressed video. Video images that have been processed to reduce the amount of bandwidth needed to capture the necessary information so that the information can be sent over a telephone network.

Computer-based patient record (CPR). A compilation in electronic form of individual patient information that resides in a system designed to provide access to complete and accurate patient data, alerts, reminders, clinical decision support systems, links to medical knowledge, and other aids.

Computer conferencing. Group communications through computers, or the use of shared computer files, remote terminal equipment, and telecommunications channels for two-way, real-time communication.

Data compression. Processing data to reduce storage and bandwidth requirements. Some compression methods result in the loss of some information, which may or may not be clinically important.

Data repository. The component of an information system that accepts, files, and stores data from a variety of sources.

DAX (digital exchange). A computerized digital cross connection that allows specific channels from high capacity lines to split out separately and be redirected.

Dedicated line. Permanent connection between two telephones or PBXs (see private branch exchange, below); the signal does not need to be switched.

Digital. Discrete signals such as those represented by bits as opposed to continuously variable analog signals. Digital technology allows communications signals to be compressed for more efficient transmission.

Digital Imaging and Communication in Medicine (DICOM). A standard for communications among medical imaging devices.

Digitizing. Conversion of analog into digital information.

Direct broadcast satellite (DBS). A satellite designed with sufficient power so that inexpensive earth stations, or downlinks, can be used for direct residential reception.

Direct digital imaging. Involves the capture of digital images so that they can be electronically transmitted.

Downlink. The path from a satellite to the Earth stations that receive its signals.

DS1. A digital carrier capable of transmitting 1.544 Mbps of electronic information. Also known as T1; the general term for a digital carrier available for high-value voice, data, or compressed video traffic.

DS3. A carrier of 45 Mbps bandwidth. One DS3 (also known as T3) channel can carry 28 DS1 channels.

Duplex. A transmission system allowing data to be transmitted in both directions simultaneously.

Earth station. The ground equipment, including a dish and other electronics needed to receive and/or transmit satellite telecommunications signals.

Electronic data interchange (EDI). The sending and receiving of data directly between trading partners without paper or human intervention.

Encryption. The rearrangement of the "bit" stream of a previously digitally encoded signal in a systematic fashion to make it unrecognizable until restored by the necessary authorization key. This technique is used for securing information transmitted over a communication channel with the intent of excluding all other than the authorized receivers from interpreting the message.

Equal access. Ability to choose between the different long-distance carriers.

Fiber distributed data interface (FDDI). A high-speed fiber optic network which has state-of-the-art bandwidth.

Fiber optics. Hair-thin, flexible glass rods encased in cables that use light to transmit audio, video, and data signals.

Film digitizer. A device that allows scanning of existing static images so that the images can be stored, manipulated, or transmitted in digital form.

Filmless radiology. Use of devices that replace film by acquiring digital images and related patient information and transmit, store, retrieve, and display them electronically.

Firewall. Computer hardware and software that block unauthorized communications between an institution's computer network and external networks.

Frame Relay. A streamlined process of sending and acknowledging transmitted packets of data which improves the rate of data transfer compared to previous transmission protocols.

Freeze-frame (Slow scan). A method of transmitting still images over standard telephone lines at a rate of one every 8 to 30 seconds.

Frequency. The rate at which an electromagnetic signal alternates, reported in Hertz.

Full duplex. A communication channel over which both transmission and reception are possible at the same time.

Full-motion video. A standard video signal requiring 6MHz (megahertz) in analog format and 45Mbps when encoded digitally.

Half-duplex. A communication channel over which both transmission and reception are possible, but only in one direction at a time.

Hardware. Physical equipment used in data processing, as opposed to computer programs and associated documentation.

Hard wired. A communication link that permanently connects two devices.

Health Care Information Infrastructure (HCII). A subset of the National Information Infrastructure (see below).

Health Level-7 Data Communications Protocol (HL-7). Defines standards for transmitting billing, hospital census, order entries, and other health-related information.

Hertz. A measure of the number of complete cycles made by an analog signal in a given time period.

High-definition television (HDTV). An advanced television system that produces video images as clear as high-quality photographs.

High Performance Computing and Communications program (HPCC). A federal, coordinated, interagency research and development effort designed to accelerate the availability and utilization of the next generation of high performance computers and networks.

Image processing. Use of algorithms to modify data representing an image, usually to improve diagnostic interpretation.

Independent telephone company. A local exchange carrier that is not part of the BOCs (Bell Operating Companies, see above), often cooperative in rural areas.

Informatics. The application of computer science and information science to the management and processing of data, information, and knowledge.

Integrated circuit. A solid state microcircuit consisting of interconnected semiconductor elements diffused into a single device.

Integrated services digital network (ISDN). A digital telecommunications technology that allows for the integrated transmission of voice, data, and video; a protocol for high-speed digital transmission.

Interexchange carrier (IXC). Also known as a long-distance carrier, a telephone company that carries long-distance calls.

Interface. The boundary between two hardware or software systems across which data are transferred.

Internet. The largest international computer network, linking computers and computer networks from colleges and universities, government agencies, institutions, and commercial organizations worldwide.

Leased lines (Dedicated lines). Lines rented from a telephone company for the exclusive use of a customer.

Local access transport area (LATA). Local telephone service areas created by the divestiture of the Regional Bell Operating Companies (RBOCs, see below) formerly associated with AT&T.

Local area networks (LANs). Private networks that facilitate the sharing of information and computer resources by members of a specific group.

Local exchange carrier (LEC). Carrier providing local services to customers within a LATA (see above).

Medical informatics. The combination of computer science, information science, and medicine designed to assist in the management and processing of data to support the delivery of health care.

Message switching. A message (image or text) divided into many parts that are then transmitted separately to the receiver where they are put back together to form the message.

Microwave. High-frequency radiowaves used for point-to-point communication of audio, video, and data signals; its spectrum is generally above 2 GHz (gigahertz).

Modem. A modulator/demodulator, this device converts digital information into analog form for transmission over a telecommunications channel and reconverts it to digital form at the point of reception.

Multiplexing. Combination of many low-capacity communications channels into one high-capacity communications channel by interleaving the various channels in discrete time or frequency slices.

Narrowband. A telecommunications medium that uses (relatively) low-frequency signals, not exceeding 1.544 Mbps.

National Information Infrastructure (NII). The integration of hardware, software, and skills that will make it easy and affordable to connect people with each other, with computers, and with a vast array of services and information resources.

Network. A set of nodes, points, or locations connected by means of data, voice, and video communications for the purpose of exchange.

Node. A branching or exchange point for networks.

Open system. A system that permits connection to a variety of other systems or technologies.

Optical character recognition (OCR). Automated scanning and conversion of printed characters to computer-based text.

Packet. A short block of data containing information on its source, content, and destination that is transferred in a packet switched network.

Packet switched network (PSN). Transmitted data broken into small packets so that each can be sent over a different route if there is extensive network traffic.

Packet switching. The process of transmitting digital information by means of addressed packets so that a channel is occupied only during the transmission of the packet.

Peripheral equipment. In a data processing system, any equipment, distinct from the central processing unit, that may provide the system with outside communication or additional facilities.

Picture archiving and communications system (PACS). A system that acquires, transmits, stores, retrieves, and displays digital images and related patient information from a variety of imaging sources and communicates the information over a network.

Pixel. The smallest displayable area on a computer screen; the fundamental picture element of a digital image.

Private branch exchange (PBX). A private telephone exchange that serves a particular organization and has connections to the public telephone network.

Point-to-point. Internal telephone systems located on the premises of many large offices.

Public switched telephone network (PSTN). The public telephone network.

Real time. The capture, processing, and presentation of data at the time the data is originated.

Regional Bell Operating Company (RBOC). One of the seven regional companies formed by the AT&T divestiture.

Repeater. A bidirectional device used to amplify or regenerate signals.

Resolution. Spatial resolution is the ability to distinguish between adjacent structures. Contrast resolution is the ability to distinguish between shades of gray.

Routing. The assignment of a communication path.

Rural area networks (RANs). Shared-usage networks, configured to include a wide range of users in rural communities, such as educational, health, and business entities.

Satellite. An electronics retransmission device serving as a repeater, placed in orbit for the purpose of receiving and retransmitting electromagnetic signals.

Signaling System 7 (SS7). A recent development in control systems for the public telephone network making telephone call processing faster and more efficient and making more services available to consumers.

Slow scan video. A device that transmits and receives still video pictures over a narrow telecommunications channel.

Store-and-forward. Transmission of static images or audio-video clips to a remote data storage device, from which they can be retrieved by a medical practitioner for review and consultation at any time, obviating the need for the simultaneous availability of the consulting parties and reducing transmission costs due to low bandwidth requirements.

Structured data entry. A data collection technique that constrains the language and format of clinical descriptions for the purpose of ensuring uniform, unambiguous, interchangeable messages.

Switch. A mechanical or solid state device that opens or closes circuits, changes operating parameters, or selects paths or circuits on a space or time division basis.

Switched line. Communication link for which the physical path, established by dialing, may vary with each use.

Switched network. A type of system where each user has a unique address that allows the network to connect any two points directly.

Synchronous transmission. The process by which bits are transmitted at a fixed rate with the transmitter and receiver synchronized, eliminating the need for start/stop elements, thus providing greater efficiency.

T1. See DS1.

T3. See DS3.

Tariffs. Price structures for communication facilities set forth by federal or local governments, intended to allow telephone companies (LATA, see local access transport area, above) a fair rate of return on their capital investments.

T-carrier. Series of transmission systems using pulse code modulation technology at various channel capacities and bit rates to send digital information over telephone lines or other transmission medium.

Telecommunications. The use of wire, radio, optical, or other electromagnetic channels to transmit or receive signals for voice, data, and video communications.

Teleconferencing. Interactive electronic communication between two or more people at two or more sites, which make use of voice, video, and/or data transmission systems.

Teleconsultation. Audio, video, or other electronic consultation between two or more geographically separated clinicians.

Telediagnosis. The detection of a disease by evaluating data transmitted to a receiving station from instruments monitoring a distant patient.

Telematics. The use of computer-based information processing in telecommunications and the use of telecommunications to allow computers to transfer programs and data to one another.

Telemedicine. The use of electronic and telecommunications technologies to provide and support health care when distance separates the participants.

Telementoring. The use of audio, video, and other telecommunications and electronic information processing technologies to provide individual guidance or instruction, for example, involving a consultant guiding a distant clinician in a new medical procedure.

Telemonitoring. The use of audio, video, and other telecommunications and electronic information processing technologies to monitor patient status at a distance.

Telepresence. The use of robotic and other devices that allow a person (e.g., a surgeon) to perform a task at a remote site by manipulating instruments (e.g., lasers or dental handpieces) and receiving sensory information or feedback (e.g., pressure akin to that created by touching a patient) that creates a sense of being present at the remote site and allows a satisfactory degree of technical performance (e.g., dexterity).

Teletext. A broadcasting service using several otherwise unused scanning lines (vertical blanking intervals) between frames of TV pictures to transmit information from a central database to receiving television sets.

Terrestrial carrier. A telecommunications transmission system using land-based facilities.

Throughput. The amount of data that can be transmitted over a network in a given period of time.

Tie line. A leased or dedicated telephone circuit provided by common carriers that links two points together without using the switched telephone network (see trunk, below).

Transmission control protocol/Internet protocol (TCP/IP). A communications protocol governing data exchanged on the Internet.

Transmission speed. The speed at which information passes over the line; defined in either bits per second (bps) or baud (see above).

Transponder. A microwave repeater (receiver and transmitter) in a satellite that receives signals being sent from Earth, amplifies them, and sends them back down to Earth for reception purposes.

Trunk. A large-capacity, long-distance channel used by common carriers to transfer information between its customers.

Twisted pair. The most prevalent type of medium in PSTN's (public switched telephone network, see above) local loops, insulated copper wires are wrapped around each other to cancel the effects of electrical noise. It can transmit voice, data, and low-grade video.

Uplink. The path/link from a transmitting Earth station to the satellite.

Validity. The extent to which an observed situation reflects the true situation.

Video conferencing. Real-time, usually two-way transmission of digitized video images between two or more locations.

Video frame grabber. A device that converts an analog video signal into a set of digital values.

Virtual circuit. Packet switched network facilities that give the appearance of an actual end-to-end circuit.

Virtual reality. A computer-based technology for simulating visual, auditory, and other sensory aspects of complex environments.

Voice grade channel. A telephone circuit of sufficient bandwidth to carry signals in the voice frequency range of 300 to 3,400 Hertz.

Voice switching. An electrical technique for opening and closing a circuit in response to the presence or absence of sound.

Wide area network (WANs). Data communication networks that provide long-haul connectivity between separate networks located in different geographic areas.

Wide area telephone service (WATS). A telephone service with a flat rate for measured bulk-rate, long-distance services provided on an incoming or outgoing basis.

World Wide Web (WWW). Internet system for worldwide hypertext linking of multimedia documents.

Workstation. A functional grouping of computer hardware and software (e.g., monitor, keyboard, hard drive) for individual uses such as word, information, and image processing.

ABBREVIATIONS

AHCPR	Agency for Health Care Policy and Research
AHEC	Area Health Education Center
AMA	American Medical Association
AMIA	American Medical Informatics Association
ANSI	American National Standards Institute
ARPA	Advanced Research Projects Agency, DOD
ASCII	American Standard Code for Information Interchange
ATA	American Telemedicine Association
ATM	Asynchronous transfer mode
BOC	Bell Operating Companies
CATV	Cable television
CD-ROM	Compact disk, read-only memory

CODEC	Coder-decoder
CPR	Computer-based patient record
CPU	Central processing unit
DBS	Direct broadcast satellite
DHHS	Department of Health and Human Services
DICOM	Digital Imaging and Communications in Medicine
DOD	Department of Defense
DVA	Department of Veterans Affairs
EDI	Electronic data interchange
HCFA	Health Care Financing Administration
HIS	Hospital Information System
HL-7	Health Level-7 Data Communications Protocol
HPCC	High Performance Computing and Communications
IOM	Institute of Medicine
ISDN	Integrated services digital network
JCAHO	Joint Commission on Accreditation of Healthcare Organizations
LAN	Local area network
LDC	Long distance carrier
LEC	Local exchange carrier
MRI	Magnetic Resonance Imaging
NAS	National Academy of Sciences
NASA	National Aeronautics and Space Administration
NIH	National Institutes of Health
NII	National Information Infrastructure
NIST	National Institute of Standards and Technology
NLM	National Library of Medicine
NRC	National Research Council
NSF	National Science Foundation
ORHP	Office of Rural Health Policy
OTA	Office of Technology Assessment

PACS	Picture archiving and communications systems
PBX	Private branch exchange
PHO	Physician hospital organization
PPO	Preferred provider organization
PSN	Packet switched network
PSTN	Public switched telephone network
RAN	Rural area network
RBOC	Regional Bell Operating Company
RIS	Radiology Information System
TCP/IP	Transmission control protocol/Internet protocol
TIE	Telemedicine Information Exchange
WAN	World area network
WATS	World area telephone service
WWW	World Wide Web

C

Committee Biographies

JOHN R. BALL, M.D., J.D., is President and CEO of Pennsylvania Hospital in Philadephia. He was previously the Executive Vice President of the American College of Physicians and a Senior Policy Analyst in the White House Office of Science and Technology Policy. Dr. Ball received his bachelor's degree from Emory University and was the first graduate of the combined medical and law program at Duke University. He is a member of the Institute of Medicine and of the Society of Medical Administrators and the American Clinical and Climatological Association, and serves on the Board of Directors of the Milbank Memorial Fund.

MICKEY S. EISENBERG, M.D., Ph.D., is the Director of Emergency Medicine Service and a professor for the Department of Medicine at the University of Washington. Dr. Eisenberg earned a bachelor's degree from the University of Michigan, a medical degree from Case Western Reserve University, and a Ph.D. in Public Health and Community Medicine from the University of Washington. He is a member of the Institute of Medicine and has published widely on topics of emergency medical services and cardiac emergencies.

MELVYN GREBERMAN, M.D., M.P.H., is Associate Director for Medical Affairs in the Center for Devices and Radiologic Health's

(CDRH's) Division of Small Manufacturers Assistance, U.S. Food and Drug Administration. Dr. Greberman earned a bachelor's degree from the University of Pennsylvania, a medical degree from Hahnemann Medical College, and a M.P.H. from Johns Hopkins University. A radiologist, he has coordinated FDA/CDRH participation in national and international programs involving the development and adoption of communication standards for digital imaging with applications in teleradiology and picture archiving and communication systems. He works with organizations such as the Department of Defense, the National Cancer Institute, the Commission of the European Union, and the European Committee for Standardization and he is a member of the federal Joint Working Group on Telemedicine. He is a Captain in the U.S. Public Health Service and a Fellow of the American College of Preventive Medicine.

MICHAEL HATTWICK, M.D., is President of Woodburn Internal Medicine Associates, a private medical practice of internal and preventative medicine. Dr. Hattwick earned a bachelor's degree (cum laude) from Harvard University, a medical degree from Baylor, and an M.P.H. equivalent degree from the University of London. He is board certified in both preventative and internal medicine. Dr. Hattwick is currently a clinical assistant professor for the Departments of Medicine and Community and Family Medicine of Georgetown University School of Medicine, a Member of the Governing Council of the Virginia Chapter of the American College of Physicians, and a Trustee of the Virginia Society of Internal Medicine. Since 1978 he has been actively using computers to implement preventive medical guidelines in his clinical practice.

SUSAN D. HORN, Ph.D., is a Senior Scientist for the Institute for Clinical Outcomes Research and a professor of medical informatics ar the University of Utah School of Medicine. Dr. Horn earned a bachelor's degree from Cornell University and a Ph.D. in statistics from Stanford. She was previously on the faculty at the Johns Hopkins University. Dr. Horn and colleagues developed the Severity of Illness Index, the Computerized Severity Index, and the Ambulatory Patient Severity system. She is a statistical consultant to a number of organizations and has authored over 100 publications on statistical methods, health services research, quality of care, and related topics.

PETER O. KOHLER, M.D., is both President of and a professor in the Department of Medicine of Oregon Health Sciences University. Dr. Kohler earned a bachelor's degree (Phi Beta Kappa) from the University of Virginia and a medical degree (AOA) from Duke Medical Center. Dr. Kohler previously served as Chair of the Oregon Health Council. He is a member of the Institute of Medicine.

NINA W. MATHESON, M.L., is Director Emerita of the William H. Welch Library and Professor of Medical Information at Johns Hopkins University. She received a bachelor's degree (cum laude, Phi Beta Kappa) from the University of Washington and a M.L. (with honors) from that university's School of Librarianship. She is a Fellow of the American College of Medical Informatics and a Distinguished Member of the Medical Library Association's Academy of Health Information Professionals. She is a member of the Institute of Medicine.

DAVID B. NASH, M.D., M.B.A., is Director of the Office of Health Policy and Clinical Outcomes at Thomas Jefferson University Hospital and Associate Professor of Medicine at Jefferson Medical College. Dr. Nash earned a bachelor's degree (Phi Beta Kappa) from Vassar College, his medical degree from the University of Rochester, and his M.B.A. in Health Administration (with honors) from the University of Pennsylvania. He is board certified in internal medicine. Among other activities, Dr. Nash is Chair, Technical Advisory Group, Pennsylvania Health Care Cost Containment Council, and a consultant to the Hartford Foundation, the federal Agency for Health Care Policy and Research, and numerous pharmaceutical corporations. He is Editor-in-Chief of the *Journal of Outcomes Management* and a member of the *Medical Economics* editorial board.

JUDITH OZBOLT, Ph.D., R.N., is a professor at the University of Virginia School of Nursing where she has previously also served as the Associate Dean for Research. Dr. Ozbolt earned a B.S.N. from Duke University and a M.S. (in Medical and Surgical Nursing) and Ph.D. (in Educational Psychology) from the University of Michigan. She was a Founding Fellow of the American Institute for Medical and Biological Engineering and chaired the Priority Expert Panel on Nursing Information Systems of NIH's National Center for Nursing Research. She was also the Program Chair and Proceedings editor for the 18th Annual Symposium on Computer Applications in Medical Care (SCAMC) in 1994. She is widely published, and her book *Decision Support Systems in Nursing* was named the American Journal of Nursing's "Book of the Year" in 1990. Dr. Ozbolt is currently a member of the Board of Directors of the American Medical Informatics Association, having previously chaired their Nursing Informatics Working Group.

JAMES S. ROBERTS, M.D., is Senior Vice President of Clinical Leadership at VHA, Inc. He is also Assistant Professor of Clinical Medicine in the Department of Medicine and Psychiatry at Northwestern University Medical School. Previously, he served as Senior Vice President of the Joint Commission of Accreditation of Healthcare Organizations. Dr. Roberts earned a bachelor's degree (Phi Beta Kappa) from Washington State University and his medical degree from Washington University School of Medicine. He is on the Editorial Advisory Board for *Quality Matters*, and is widely published in a variety of clinical and research journals.

JAY H. SANDERS, M.D., was until recently Professor of Medicine and Surgery and Director of the Telemedicine Center at the Medical College of Georgia where he also held the Eminent Scholar Chair in Telemedicine. He is now President and CEO of the Global Telemedicine Group. In addition, he is a Senior Advisor to NASA on telemedicine and the President as well as a founding member of the Board of Directors of the American Telemedicine Association. Dr. Sanders earned a bachelor's degree (Phi Beta Kappa and magna cum laude) from Colgate University and his medical degree from Harvard Medical School (magna cum laude, AOA). He has spent the majority of his professional career involved in teaching, health care research, and the development of interactive telecommunications as a means of addressing the problems relating to quality, cost, and access to care. Dr. Sanders designed the telemedicine system at the Medical College of Georgia and oversaw the implementation of a statewide telemedicine system that interfaces with rural hospitals, public health facilities, correctional institutions, and ambulatory health centers. He is Senior Editor of the *Telemedicine Journal* and a Fellow of the American College of Physicians and the American College of Asthma, Allergy, and Immunology. He is a member of the FCC Telecommunications and Health Care Advisory Committee.

JOHN C. SCOTT, M.S., is President of the Center for Public Service Communications which helps domestic and international educational, scientific, and health and humanitarian organizations apply new telecommunications technologies to their programs. He serves as the Coordinator of the Congressional Ad Hoc Steering Committee on Telemedicine and Health Informatics, and he organized the Working Conference on Telemedicine Policy for the NII and co-edited their report. He co-authored the Guide to Telemedicine Programs, Projects, and Opportunities as well as the Office of Rural Health Policy's report (the result of a focus group on the Evaluation of Practitioner Receptivity to Telemedicine) *The Human Dimension of Telemedicine*. He has also participated in several international telemedicine efforts including the Persian Gulf Telemedicine Project, Disaster Telemedicine Spacebridge to Armenia and Ufa, USAID Hospital Partnership Program in the New Independent States of the Former Soviet Union, and the International Telemedicine Spacebridge Project.

JANE E. SISK, Ph.D., is a professor in the Division of Health Policy and Management at Columbia University School of Public Health. Dr. Sisk earned a B.A. (Phi Beta Kappa, magna cum laude) from Brown University, an M.A. in economics from George Washington University, and a Ph.D. in economics from McGill University. Before coming to Columbia, she directed projects at the Congressional Office of Technology Assessment as Senior Associate and Project Director in the Health Program. She has also served as President of the International Society of Technology Assessment in Health Care (for which she was also a Founding Member). Dr. Sisk is currently a member of the New York State Task Force on Clinical Guidelines and Medical Technology Assessment and serves on the editorial boards of *Health Services Research* and the *International Journal of Technology Assessment in Health Care*.

PAUL C. TANG, M.D., is Medical Director of Information Systems at Northwestern Memorial Hospital, and Associate Professor of Medicine at Northwestern University Medical School. He is responsible for the planning and implementation of a new clinical information system for the health system, while maintaining his clinical and teaching responsibilities at the medical school. Dr. Tang received his B.S. and M.S. (Phi Beta Kappa, Tau Beta Pi) in Electrical Engineering from Stanford University, and his M.D. (Alpha Omega Alpha) from University of California at San Francisco. He is board certified in internal medicine. Dr. Tang directed research on physician workstations at Hewlett-Packard Laboratories for 10 years. He is chairman of the Computer-based Patient Record Institute (CPRI) and a Board member of the American Medical Informatics Association. He is a Fellow of the American College of Medical Informatics and the American College of Physicians.

ERIC TANGALOS, M.D., is an Associate Professor of Medicine at the Mayo Clinic. He attended the University of Michigan as an undergraduate before going on to obtain a medical degree from Loyola University's Stritch School of Medicine. Dr. Tangalos has served as Vice Chair of the Mayo Foundation Communication Committee. He was Course Director of the "First Mayo Telemedicine Symposium" and Co-Director for the "Second International Conference on the Medical Aspects of Telemedicine." He is a founding Board Member of the American Telemedicine Association and Immediate Past President of the American Medical Directors Association. He currently serves on the Editorial Boards for the international *Journal of Telemedicine and Telecare* and its stateside counterpart, the *Telemedicine Journal*. Dr. Tangalos is also a member of the FCC Telecommunications and Health Care Advisory Committee.

Index

A

Academic medical centers, 3, 18, 44.
  See also individual facilities
Acceptability of telemedicine, 8, 152,
  206
Acceptance of telemedicine. *See also*
  Patient and clinician perspectives;
  Patient satisfaction data
  documented benefits and 80–81
  health care restructuring and, 4, 81–
  82
  human factors and, 73–82
  patient, 80, 147
  payment concerns, 81
  professional, 79–80
Access to care
  barriers, 173–174
  definitions and concepts, 8, 32,
  175–176, 205
  and development of telemedicine, 2,
  53
  health information, 174
  and quality of care, 192
  questions about, 12–13, 176–179,
  205
  telecommunications rates and, 85
Advanced Research Projects Agency,
  120 n.2, 239

Agamemnon, 34
Agency for Health Care Policy and
  Research, 22, 117
Allina Healthcare Systems, 52
Ambulatory care clinics, 38–39
American College of Physicians, 22
American College of Radiology, 72
American Medical Association, 98,
  103, 106
American Medical Informatics
  Association, 41
American National Standards Institute,
  69
American Society for Testing and
  Materials, 69
Americans with Disabilities Act, 103
Anesthesiology, 38
Annals of Internal Medicine, 154
Appropriateness of care, 12, 108, 110,
  123, 166–167, 175–176, 178
Automated telephone-based services,
  45, 129–130

B

Bell, Alexander Graham, 35
Bell Operating Companies, 240

Blue Cross and Blue Shield
    Association, 22, 109
Bowman Gray, 44
Brigham and Women's Hospital, 44
Business plan/project management
    plan, 3, 6, 148–149, 155, 202–
    203

C

Cable television
    definition, 240
    rates, 85
    telemedicine applications, 38–39
California, confidentiality of medical
    records, 92
Cameras, digital, 50, 56
Center for Devices and Radiological
    Health, 113–114
Center for Health Policy Research,
    122–124, 126, 132
Center for Health Services Research,
    122
Cleveland State University, 129–130
Clinical applications of telemedicine.
    See also specific applications
    categories, 29–30
    central/consulting site, 30, 58–59
    definition, 28
    diffusion of, 194
    and evaluation, 116–117, 141
    examples, 29, 31
    remote site, 30, 58–59
Clinical decision support systems, 58
Clinical information systems, 58, 241
Clinical practice guidelines, 22, 98
Clinical Telemedicine Cooperative
    Group, 124, 133, 135–136
Clinicians. See Patient and clinician
    perspectives
Cochrane Collaboration, 22
CODEC, 50, 241
Colorado
    confidentiality of medical records,
    92
    prison telemedicine program, 46
    teleradiology standards, 100

Columbia University Health Sciences
    Division (New York), 237
Community effects of telemedicine, 9,
    163
Comparison (control) group, 6, 150–
    151, 198, 203
Compressed video, 42, 241
Computed axial tomography, 42, 56
Computer Aided Diagnosis (CADx)
    Working Group, 115
Computer conferencing, 241
Computer systems
    architecture, 239
    compatibility issues, 68–69, 72–73,
    77, 195
    millennium problem, 73
    multimedia, 78
    peripheral equipment, 50, 246
    regulation as medical devices, 114–
    115
    standards, 98, 122–123
    workstations, 35, 49, 50, 63, 77,
    78, 115, 250
Conferencing. See Computer
    conferencing; Teleconferencing
Confidentiality, 83, 92, 95, 101, 102,
    196. See also Privacy
Continuous quality improvement, 154–
    155, 166
Costs and cost-effectiveness of care.
    See also Economic analyses;
    Payment for services
    data transmission technology and,
    66
    definition, 8
    emergency services network, 53
    prison telemedicine, 46–47
    technology, 68, 78, 182, 186
    teleconsultations, 52, 53
    transportation issues, 180
Costs of technologies, 2, 39–40
Credentialing, 95–96
Croatia, 131

D

Data
    bits, 66, 240

collection instruments, 133, 161,
  171, 178, 187, 188, 207, 240
confidentiality, 102
quality issues, 123
Data security, 102. *See also* Privacy
  auditing and tracking programs, 107
  authentication procedures, 107, 240
  authorization procedures, 107
  confidentiality agreements, 101
  defined, 102
  encryption, 107, 243
  firewalls, 107, 243
  systems, 101, 106–107
Data transmission
  asynchronous, 239
  bandwidth, 61, 63–65, 240
  by coaxial cable, 65–66, 241
  compressed, 42, 67, 241, 242
  costs, 66
  digital/digitizing, 66–67
  packet switching, 67, 246
  real-time, 65, 76, 129, 246
  standards, 72, 123
  store-and-forward technologies, 16–
    17, 50, 65, 77, 247
  synchronous, 247
  by telephone, 65
  T1 (DS1) lines, 62, 63, 242
Demonstration projects. *See also*
    specific projects
  diversity, 41
  evaluation, 86, 118, 124, 135, 148
  funding, 85, 113
  HCFA, 109
  policies, 83–84, 85, 197
  professional education, 39–40
  rural economic development, 86
  sustainability, 53, 74, 75, 118, 136,
    138–139
Department of Commerce, 86, 117
Department of Defense
  evaluation of telemedicine, 24, 117,
    120–121, 130–131, 142, 204
  Hospital Information System, 62, 63
  projects, 39, 40; *see also* Military
    telemedicine
Department of Health and Human
    Services, 86, 106, 117, 199–200.
    See also Health Care Financing

Administration; National Library
  of Medicine; Office of Rural
  Health Policy
Department of Health, Education and
  Welfare, 39
Department of Veterans Affairs, 40,
  89, 117, 121–122, 204. *See also*
  VA facilities and services
Dermatology. *See* Teledermatology
Dialysis center, 49, 51
Digital images/imaging
  conventional images compared to,
    127–129
  direct, 242
  software, 86
  store-and-forward technologies, 16–
    17
Digital Imaging and Communication in
  Medicine (DICOM) standard,
  72, 242
Digital Imaging Network Project, 39
Digitizing, 42, 66–67, 242
Distance medicine, 28
Documentation of methods and results,
  6, 154, 191, 202, 203
Drew Health Foundation, 51

                            E

East Carolina University School of
  Medicine, 47
Eastern Montana Telemedicine
  Network, 230–231
Eastern Oregon Human Services
  Consortium, 47–48
Eastern Oregon State College, 48
Economic analyses. *See also* Costs and
    cost-effectiveness of care
  billed charges, 182–183
  capital costs, 181–182
  conceptual challenges, 183–184
  cost-benefit analysis, 181, 192–193
  cost-effectiveness analysis, 181
  decision rules, 184–186
  definitions and concepts, 32, 180–
    183, 205–206
  discounting, 182
  dynamic simulation model, 134–135

level and perspective, 179–180
needs, 128, 198
patient vs provider perspectives, 148, 175
principles, 138
productivity assessment, 128
questions about, 13, 184, 185, 206
real-options vs net-present-value, 135
sensitivity analysis, 154, 184
teledermatology, 43 n.6
variable costs, 182
ECRI (formerly Emergency Care Research Institute), 22
Education and training
networks, 47
objectives and effects of telemedicine, 9, 153, 172–173
patient, 29
professional, 29, 36, 39–40, 42–43, 47, 48, 52, 66, 87, 88
radiology and pathology images, 42–43
technical, 58–59
Electrocardiograms, 38, 45, 51
Electronic housecall, 19, 21, 45–46
Electronic mail, 46, 77
Emergency services
911, 1, 36, 45
evaluation of, 167–168
image interpretation, 127–128
network, 52–53
telemetry, 38
Emory University, 44
Evaluation of telemedicine. *See also* Research strategies
for access to care, 8, 12–13, 32, 173–179, 192, 205, 207
and acceptance, 8, 80–81, 205–207
assessment studies, 119, 128
business plan/project management plan, 3, 6, 148–149, 155, 202–203
categories, 118, 119, 134
challenges, 4–5, 10, 22, 116, 118, 183–184, 197–199
and continuous improvement, 154–155, 166
controlled vocabulary, 191–192

cooperation among institutions and individuals, 125, 198–199
criteria, 8, 32, 163, 191–192
definitions, 30–33
documentation of methods and results, 6, 154, 191, 202, 203
domains, 147, 162–163
economic analysis, 8, 13, 32, 47, 128, 134–135, 148, 156, 179–186, 192–193, 205–207
effectiveness and cost-effectiveness, 32, 132–136
elements, 144–154, 202–204
feasibility determinations, 140, 142–144, 191
federal role, 7, 117–118, 136, 141–142, 199–200, 204; *see also individual agencies*
formative, 134, 193
frameworks, 2, 5–7, 17–18, 30–31, 86, 118–126, 137–161, 162, 173–174, 200–207
human factors assessment, 74–75, 155, 164, 195–196
importance, 137, 207–208
improvement of, 199–200, 207
institutional, 147
lack of evaluation, 17, 116–117
level of, 6, 146–148, 164, 179–180, 203
literature, 7, 126–127
needs assessment, 78–79
objectives, 12, 119, 136, 139–141, 145–146, 154
obstacles to, 118, 132, 137, 138, 184
patient and clinician perspectives, 14–15, 148, 186–190, 206
planning for, 138–144, 156, 201–202
policy-related variables, 84, 87
pooling of information, 124–125
population-directed, 32–33, 47, 164–165, 176, 178
principles, 5, 24–25, 137–138, 155, 200–201
priority-setting, 141–142
private-sector role, 7
processes of care, 6, 13, 151

project description, 144–145, 203
purpose, 17, 116, 194
for quality of care, 8, 11, 32, 128,
  163, 165–173, 205–207
and reimbursement for services,
  117, 123–124, 166
resource issues, 142
strategies; *see* Research strategies
summative, 134
system/societal, 147–148, 179
telecardiology, 190
teledermatology, 125, 128–129,
  131–132, 143, 144–145, 147
telepsychiatry, 45, 147, 162, 181
teleradiology, 44, 116, 124, 127–
  128, 147, 168

F

Fair Health Information Practices Act,
  105
Fax machines, 77
Federal Communications Commission,
  85
Federal Food, Drug, and Cosmetic Act,
  114
Federation of State Medical Boards,
  94–95
Florida, licensure laws, 90
Fluoroscopy, 38
Food and Drug Administration,
  medical device regulation, 57–
  58, 86, 113–115
Fort Detrick Army Medical Research
  and Materiel Command, 120
Freestanding specialty groups, 18

G

Gastroenterology applications, 47 n.7
General Accounting Office, 87
George Washington University, 40
Georgia, telemedicine reimbursements,
  109
Grants, federal, 41, 47–48, 52, 229–238
Greater Oregon Behavioral Health,
  Inc., 48

H

Haiti, 131
Hardware. *See also* Computer systems;
  specific devices
compatibility, 77, 241
definition, 244
problems, 75–76
standards, 3, 69–72, 82, 98
Harvard Community Health Plan, 101
Health care administration,
  telemedicine applications in, 29,
  52, 62, 63
Health Care Financing Administration
  (HCFA) (DHHS)
evaluation of telemedicine, 24, 117,
  122, 123–124, 125, 126, 132–
  133, 134, 140–141, 199–200
grants, 236–237
payment policies, 107–109, 112,
  123–124
Health Care Information Infrastructure
  (HCII), 244
Health care institutions, telemedicine
  capacity, 20
Health care restructuring, 4, 81–82,
  105, 173, 199
Health care technologies, assessment
  of, 22–24
Health Information Applications
  Working Group, 74, 86
Health insurance programs, privacy
  issues, 103
Health Level Seven (HL7) standard,
  69–72, 244
Health maintenance organizations
  (HMOs), 20, 51, 112, 159. *See
  also* Managed care
Health Security Act of 1993, 105
Health Services Research, 154
Healthspan, 52
Hewlett-Packard, 49
High Performance Computing and
  Communications program, 86,
  244
High Plains Rural Health Network,
  232
Hippocratic Oath, 103

Home health options, 1, 44–46, 168, 184
Human factors in telemedicine
  and acceptance of telemedicine, 73–82
  assessment, 74–75, 155, 164, 195–196
  cultural and socioeconomic, 79–82
  needs and preference assessment, 78–79
  equipment-related problems, 75–76
  incorporation in existing practice, 76–78
  recognition of, 74–75

I

Image processing, 244
Implementation of telemedicine, 138, 152, 155
Indiana, licensure laws, 90
Information Infrastructure Task Force Committee on Applications, 74, 86
Information technologies, 28, 60–61. *See also* Clinical information systems
Infrastructure. *See* Technical infrastructure
Integrated services digital network (ISDN), 67, 244
Interactive video, 1, 16, 19, 28, 36, 38, 40–41, 48, 49, 50, 53
Interactive voice response systems, 45
Intergovernmental Health Policy Program, 87
International Standards Organizations, 69
Internet, 41, 46, 80, 125, 182, 244–245, 249. *See also* World Wide Web
Interstate telemedicine, 3, 83, 89–95
Iowa
  Health System Telemedicine Demonstration, 236
  programs and initiatives, 87

J

Jackson Memorial Hospital, Miami, 38
Jean-Talon Hospital, 36
Johns Hopkins University, 127–128
Joint Commission on Accreditation of Healthcare Organizations, 95, 96, 103, 114
Joint Working Group on Telemedicine, 7, 24, 40, 86, 119, 120, 162, 200
Journal of the American Medical Association, 154
Journals. *See also specific journals*
  on-line, 20
  peer-review process, 20
  research documentation guidance, 154

K

Kaiser Permanente of Southern California, 22
Kansas
  Board of Healing Arts, 91
  telemedicine reimbursements, 109
Kentucky Telecare, 232–233

L

Learning curve, 172
Legislation. *See also* Medicare; Payment for services; *individual topics*
  malpractice, 100
  medical device, 114
  national licensure, 93–94
  privacy/confidentiality-related, 105–106
  telecommunications, 66, 84–85, 132 n.5
Liability. See Malpractice liability
Licensure, professional
  credentialing, 95–96
  by endorsement, 91
  issues, 3, 81, 83, 92
  options, 93–95, 105
  policies, current, 89–91, 196

Literature
   buyers guide, 56
   evaluation research, 116, 126, 149–150
   outcome measures, 171
   searches, 50
   telemedicine applications, 40, 75
Lockheed Company, 39
Logan Airport, Boston, 38
Louisiana, licensure laws, 90
Lytton Gardens Health Care Center, 49–51

M

Macedonia, 131
Magnetic resonance imaging, 42
Malpractice liability
   data security and, 106
   issues, 3, 83, 97–99
   options, 99–100
   organizational, 99
   policies, current, 96–97
Mammography, 113, 124, 128
Managed care
   cost effectiveness, 180
   payment policies, 108, 111
   quality-of-care assessments, 163, 164–165
   and professional opportunities, 174–175
   telemedicine in, 3, 9, 18, 20, 32–33, 52–53
Mary Imogene Bassett Hospital, 231
Maryland
   confidentiality of medical records, 92
   trauma center, 89
Massachusetts General Hospital, 38
MDTV (Mountain Doctor Television), 229–230, 236–237
md/tv, inc., 49
Medica, 52
Medicaid, 180
Medical Advanced Technology Management Office, 120
Medical College of Georgia, 133–134, 236

Medical Device Amendments of 1976, 114
Medical devices
   definition, 114
   regulation of, 57–58, 86, 113–115
   safety evaluation, 118
Medical Outcomes Study, 189
Medical Outcomes Trust, 22
Medical Privacy in the Age of New Technologies Act, 105
Medical Records Confidentiality Act, 105
Medicare, 3, 42, 43, 81, 102–103, 107–108, 109, 111, 112, 117, 134, 141, 196
Memorial University of Newfoundland, 39–40
Miami Fire Department, 38
Microscopy, 38
Microwave transmission, 34, 38, 66, 245
Mid-Nebraska Telemedicine Network, 231
Military telemedicine
   evaluation of, 120–121, 130–131, 147, 168, 200
   initiatives, 43, 56–57
   interstate activities, 89
   payment policies, 107
Minnesota
   confidentiality of medical records, 92
   telemedicine initiatives, 52
Missouri Telemedicine Network, 233
Mt. Sinai School of Medicine, New York City, 38–39
Multiorganization medical consortia, 18

N

National Academy of Engineering, 38
National Academy of Sciences
   Computer Science and Telecommunications Board, 102
National Aeronautics and Space Administration, 39

National Association of Insurance
  Commissioners, 106
National Commission on Quality
  Assurance, 95
National Electrical Manufacturers
  Association, 72
National Information Infrastructure, 2,
  20–21, 60–61, 86, 245
National Institute of Standards and
  Technology, 117
National Library of Medicine (DHHS),
  2
  evaluation of telemedicine, 117,
    129, 142, 199
  Grateful Med, 24
  literature on telemedicine, 40
  Loansome Doc, 24
  Medline, 20, 24
  privacy/security initiatives, 102
  real-time treatment technology
    programs, 235–236
  testbed networks, 234–235
  Uniform Medical Language System
    Metathesaurus, 192
  virtual reality, 235
  workshops/conferences on
    telemedicine, 74
National Naval Medical Center,
  Bethesda, 59, 62–63
National Telecommunications and
  Information Administration, 84–
  86, 117, 237–238
Naval Medical Center, Annapolis, 59
Nebraska programs and initiatives, 87,
  89
Networks and networking. *See also*
  specific networks
  circuit switched, 241
  communications, 72
  definition, 61, 245–246
  packet switched, 246
  peer, 48
  privacy and confidentiality issues,
    104
  professional education, 47, 48
  public switched telephone (PSTN),
    246
  rural area, 52, 135, 247
  specialty consultation, 135

switched, 247
teleradiology, 44
wide area, 250
Neurological applications, 36, 47 n.7
Nevada, licensure laws, 90
New York, confidentiality of medical
  records, 92
Norfolk State Hospital, 36
Norman, Donald, 73–74
North Carolina
  Central Prison Telemedicine Project,
    46–47
  Emergency Consult Network, 168
  programs and initiatives, 87, 167–168
Nurse practitioners, 39, 170, 172–173
Nurses, 18–19
  emergency services, 53
  telephone advisory services, 45
Nursing homes, telemedicine
  applications in, 38, 49–51

O

Office of Rural Health Policy (DHHS)
  evaluation of telemedicine, 117,
    135, 140, 142
  grants, 41, 47–48, 52, 229–233
  role in present study, 24
  survey of telemedicine use, 20
  workshops and conferences, 74–75
Oklahoma County, Oklahoma, City-
  County Health Department, 237
Oregon
  ED-NET, 48, 88
  evaluation research, 129, 131–132
  Health Sciences University, 48, 129,
    131–132
  malpractice legislation, 100
  telepsychiatry program, 47–49, 66
Outcomes of care, measures, 6, 9, 11,
  32, 128, 134, 146, 152–153,
  163, 170–171, 176, 192, 205,
  207

P

Pacemaker surveillance, 45
Pacific Bell, 49

Paramedics, 38
Patient and clinician perspectives
    methods and focus, 188
    quality of care, 19, 186–187; *see
        also* Patient satisfaction
    questions, 14, 189–190, 206
Patient care, telemedicine applications,
    29, 31, 38
Patient information systems
    applications of telemedicine, 31, 50
    benefits and risks, 104
    compatibility, 72–73, 77
    computer-based patient record
        (CPR), 58, 86, 99, 103–104,
        121, 171, 204, 207, 241
    and evaluation of telemedicine, 7,
        160–161, 171, 204
    Health Level Seven (HL7) standard,
        69–72
    and malpractice liability, 99
    privacy and confidentiality, 3–4, 78,
        83, 92, 95, 99, 101, 103–106,
        196
    security measures, 101, 105–106
    utilization, 20
    Veterans Administration, 121
Patient satisfaction data, 8, 14, 147,
    163, 176, 186–187, 188, 206
Patients, telemedicine use, 19
Payment for services. *See also*
        Medicare
    and acceptability of telemedicine, 81
    capitation payment/fixed budget,
        108, 111–112, 166, 171–172,
        180, 183
    commercial organizations, 113
    copayments, 112
    demonstration projects and, 113
    evaluation research and, 117
    fee-for-service, 43 n.6, 107–110,
        111, 166, 180, 196
    per case or other bundled methods,
        110–111, 171–172, 183
    policies, 83, 196
    radiology, 3, 42, 43
Pennsylvania
    Keystone State Desktop Medical
        Conferencing Network, 238
    licensure laws, 90

Physician hospital organizations
    (PHOs), 20
Physician Payment Review
    Commission, 109
Physicians. *See also* Human factors in
        telemedicine; Patient and
        clinician perspectives;
        Practitioners
    income concerns, 18
    information technologies relevant
        to, 63
    surplus, 18
    use of telemedicine, 19–20
Picasso, 57
Picture archiving and communications
    system (PACS), 42, 43, 57, 62,
    63, 114–115, 246
Policy issues. *See* Telemedicine policy
Postsurgical monitoring, 49–51
Practitioner-patient relationships, 18
Practitioners
    databases, 92, 135
    perceptions of telemedicine, 14–15
Preferred provider organizations
    (PPOs), 20
Prison telemedicine projects, 43 n.6,
    46–47, 88, 89, 107
Privacy. *See also* Confidentiality; Data
        security
    informational, 101–102
    issues, 3–4, 83, 101, 103–105, 196
    options, 105–106
    policies, current, 102–103
    technical and administrative
        options, 106–107
Processes of care, 11, 31, 167, 168–
    170
Psychiatry. *See* Telepsychiatry
Public health, telemedicine applications
    in, 29

                    Q

Quality of care
    definitions and concepts, 8, 32,
        165–168, 205
    educational effects of telemedicine,
        172–173

outcome measures, 167–168, 170–171
patient risk and, 171–172
patient satisfaction measures, 163, 206–207
practitioner concerns, 19
process measures, 168–170
questions about, 11, 168–172
severity of illness and, 171–172, 206
teledermatology, 43 n.6
types of problems, 166
volume-outcome hypothesis, 173

R

Radio News, 35–36, 37
Radiology. *See* Teleradiology
Radiotelemetry, 38
Rapid City Regional Hospital, 230
REACH-TV, 231–232, 237
Regional Bell Operating Companies, 49, 52, 246
Regulation of medical devices, 57–58, 86, 113–115
Research, telemedicine applications in, 29, 36
Research strategies. *See also* Evaluation of telemedicine
    administrative processes, 6, 151–152, 203
    automated telephone-based strategies, 129–130
    clinical aspects, 6, 13, 119, 120, 141, 146, 147, 151, 155, 156, 167, 203
    clinical practice study, 160
    comparison (control) group, 6, 150–151, 198, 203
    data collection, 161, 171, 178
    with deployed troops, 130–131
    design, 6, 7, 10, 119, 139, 142, 143, 149–150, 155, 156–161, 164, 204
    digital vs conventional images, 127–129
    effectiveness trial, 159, 160
    efficacy, 157, 159

event/problem logs, 152, 155
experimental design, 157, 159, 161, 204
experimental group, 6, 150–151, 203
large simple trials, 159
literature on, 149–150, 156–157, 171
nonexperimental, 161, 204
objectives, 6, 145–146, 162
outcome measures, 6, 9, 11, 32, 128, 134, 146, 152–153, 163, 165–166, 167, 168–169, 170–171, 176, 192, 203, 205
patient information systems and, 7, 160–161, 171, 204
processes of care, 11, 31, 167, 168–170
quasi-experimental, 160–161, 204
questions (research), 6, 7–9, 11–15, 119, 124, 125–126, 140, 145, 147, 162, 163–165, 168–172, 176–179, 184, 185, 189–190, 193, 199, 203, 205, 206
randomized clinical trials, 157, 159
retrospective analysis, 161, 168–169
sensitivity analysis, 5–7, 153–154, 156, 164–165, 203
technical infrastructure, 6, 151, 203
teledermatology services for rural areas, 131–132
test-of-concept, 119, 121, 126, 134, 143–144, 148, 150, 193, 201, 202
validity, 157–158, 160, 171, 191, 249
RODEO NET (Rural Options for Development and Educational Opportunities), 47–48
Rural Health Alliance Telemedicine Network, 52
Rural telemedicine
    access issues, 173
    dermatology, 131–132
    cost effectiveness, 66, 85
    effects, 9
    payment for services, 112
    psychiatry, 47–49
    radiology, 43
    utilization, 40

S

Saint Louis University School of Public Health, Missouri, 238
San Jose Medical Group, 51
Satellite systems, 66
Senate/House Ad Hoc Steering Committee on Telemedicine, 85
Sensitivity analysis
  economic, 154, 184
  research strategies, 5–7, 153–154, 156, 164–165, 203
Social security numbers, private market for, 105
Software
  evaluation tools, 125–126
  medical, regulation of, 57–58, 86, 115
Somalia, 43 n.6, 121, 131, 168
South Carolina, licensure laws, 90
South Dakota, licensure laws, 90
Space Technology Applied to Rural Papago Advanced Health Care (STARPAHC), 39
Speech therapy, 36
St. Paul Fire & Marine Insurance, 100
Standards/standardization
  of care, 97, 100
  hardware and software, 3, 69–72, 82, 98
  medical devices, 113–114
  questionnaires, 133, 161, 171, 178, 187
Stanford University Medical Center, 49–51, 129
State
  confidentiality provisions, 102, 106
  evaluation research, 118
  licensure laws, 89–90, 102, 196
  malpractice laws, 96–97
  programs and initiatives, 40, 87–89
Stethoscope, electronic, 38, 50, 56
Store-and-forward technologies, 16–17, 50, 65, 77, 129, 247
Surgeon General of the Army, 117, 120
Surgery. *See* Telesurgery
Survey of telemedicine users, 40
Switching, advanced digital, 42

T

Tactile data, 31
Technical infrastructure
  compatibility of systems, 3, 27, 67–69, 195
  costs, 182
  digital technologies, 66–67
  equipment and space configurations, 59
  information carrying capacity, 61–65
  information restructuring, 66–67
  innovations, 21
  location of units, 77
  obsolescence, 4, 72–73, 182, 197–198
  projects, 87
  service providers, services, and resources, 57
  standards for hardware and software, 3, 69–72
  technologies, 4, 35, 55–56, 59–73
  transmission media, 65–66
  user needs and circumstances and, 3, 58–59, 198
Technology training, 48
Telecardiology, 109, 190. *See also* Electrocardiograms
Telecommunications. *See also* Data transmission; Telephone communications
  costs, 2, 40, 63
  definition, 248
  evaluation of technology, 120
  evolution of, 34–35
  in health care sector, 56
  infrastructure, 88
  legislation, 66, 84–85, 132 n.5
  media, 28
  policy, 84–86
  programs, 87
  transoceanic, 38
Telecommunications Bill of 1996, 84–85
Teleconferencing
  administrative, 62, 63
  audio, 240
  clinical, 49, 62, 63
  definition, 248

educational, 20
interactive video, 16, 28, 48, 49, 62,
    63, 249
real-time, 65
store-and-forward systems, 65
workstation, 49, 62, 63
Teleconsultation
cost-effectiveness, 52
definition, 248
diagnostic, 36, 38
equipment and space
    configurations, 51, 59, 62–63
interstate licensure policies, 90, 91
and malpractice, 98
in nursing homes, 49
payment policies, 107, 109
scheduling problems, 76–77
specialist, 52
utilization, 47 n.7, 131
Teledermatology
applications, 49, 51, 131
evaluation of, 125, 128–129, 131–
    132, 143, 144–145, 147
imaging, 56, 128–129, 143
rural applications, 131–132
utilization, 43 n.6, 47 n.7
Telediagnosis, 36, 38, 99, 167, 248
Telegraph, 34–35
Telemedicine. See also Payment for
    services
applications, 1, 2–3, 7, 16–17, 19–
    20, 28–31, 40–53
context for, 18–22
definition, 1, 26–29, 248
development, 2–4, 35–40
demand for evidence of
    effectiveness, 1–2, 22–24, 109,
    116
federal projects, 39; see also
    Demonstration projects;
    individual agencies and projects
growth and diversity, 40–41, 198,
    201–202
inventory of projects, 86, 121
obstacles to use, 3–4, 53, 58–59,
    67–68, 83, 107, 108, 195–196
status, 19–21
structure of report, 33
study origins and approach, 24–26

Telemedicine Information Exchange,
    41, 125 n.3
Telemedicine Journal, 154
Telemedicine policy. See also
    Licensure, professional;
    Malpractice liability; Payment
    for services; Privacy; Regulation
    of medical devices
national communications policy
    and, 84–86
state programs and initiatives, 87–
    89
Telemedicine Research Center, 124–
    126, 129
Telemedicine Testbed, 120
Telementoring, 27, 28, 248
Telemonitoring, 27, 45, 49–51, 130,
    133 n.6, 168, 184, 248
Telepathology, 109, 116, 128
Telephone communications
advisory programs, 44–45
automated, 129–130
consultation and triage, 121
emergency 911, 1, 36, 45
evaluation of, 129–130
health risk assessment program,
    129–130
history, 35, 77
human factors in, 77
importance, 53
lines, 65
monitoring system, 130
still-image system, 57
Telepresence, 27, 248–249
Telepsychiatry, 27, 36, 38, 45, 47–49,
    65, 66, 104, 124, 147, 162, 175,
    181
Telequest, 44
Teleradiology
applications of telemedicine, 20, 36,
    38, 41–44, 121
digital image management, 39, 42,
    57
economic benefits, 181
evaluation of, 44, 116, 124, 127–
    128, 147
filmless, 43, 243
growth of, 36, 38, 40–41
image quality, 127–128

networks, 39, 44
payment for services, 3, 42, 43,
    109, 196
standards, 72, 100
workstation, 62, 63
Telesurgery, 1, 16, 86, 124
Television, 36, 37, 38. *See also* Cable
    television; Interactive video
Texas
    licensure laws, 90
    prison telemedicine program, 46, 88
Texas Tech, 47
Timeliness of care, 12–13, 128, 192
Total quality management, 166
Training effect, 153
Tripler Army Medical Center, 120

U

Uniform State Code for Telemedicine
    Licensure and Credentialing, 93
University of
    California at San Francisco, 44
    Colorado Health Sciences Center,
        122
    Iowa, 43
    Miami School of Medicine, 38
    Michigan, 133–134, 236
    Minnesota Telemedicine Project,
        233
    Nebraska, 36, 87, 89
    North Carolina at Chapel Hill, 230
    Pennsylvania, 44
    Texas Medical Branch at Galveston,
        47
    Washington, 135
Urban telemedicine
    ambulatory care clinics, 38–39
    emergency telemetric, 38
    nursing homes, 38, 49–51
U.S. Constitution
    Commerce Clause, 93
    privacy protection, 102
U.S. Indian Health Service, 39
U.S. Office of Technology Assessment,
    58, 105, 159–160, 161
U.S. Public Health Service, 39, 89
U.S. West, 52

Utah, initiatives and programs, 88
Utilization of telemedicine, 20, 40, 43
    n.6, 47 n.7, 131, 153, 166, 169–
    170, 176, 178, 207

V

VA facilities and services
    Baltimore medical center, 43, 121,
        128
    Bedford, Massachusetts, hospital,
        38
    Decentralized Hospital Computer
        Program, 43
    evaluation of telemedicine, 200
    pacemaker surveillance centers, 45
    Palo Alto medical center, 121
    San Francisco, 45
    Washington, D.C., 45
Video technologies. *See also* Interactive
    video
    full-motion, 63
    teleconferencing workstation, 62,
        63
    transmission considerations, 63–64
Virginia initiatives and programs, 88
Virtual glove, 31
Virtual reality, 86, 250
Voice mail, 77

W

WAMI Rural Telemedicine Network,
    135, 233
West Virginia, evaluation research,
    133, 134
West Virginia University, 229–230
Western Governors Association, 87,
    93–94
World Wide Web, 20, 41, 42, 46, 47,
    113 n.11, 250

X

X-rays, ship-to-shore transmission, 38.
    See also Teleradiology